Painful Conditions of the Upper Limb

What Do I Do Now? – Pain Medicine

SERIES EDITORS

Mark P. Jensen and Lynn R. Webster

Painful Conditions of the Upper Limb

Edited by
Ramon Cuevas-Trisan, MD
Associate Chief of Staff for Education & Research
West Palm Beach VA Medical Center
Riviera Beach, FL

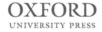

OXFORD
UNIVERSITY PRESS

Oxford University Press is a department of the University of Oxford. It furthers
the University's objective of excellence in research, scholarship, and education
by publishing worldwide. Oxford is a registered trade mark of Oxford University
Press in the UK and certain other countries.

Published in the United States of America by Oxford University Press
198 Madison Avenue, New York, NY 10016, United States of America.

© Oxford University Press 2021

Library of Congress Cataloging-in-Publication Data
Names: Cuevas-Trisan, Ramon, author.
Title: Painful conditions of the upper limb / Ramon Cuevas-Trisan.
Description: New York : Oxford University Press, [2021] |
Includes bibliographical references and index.
Identifiers: LCCN 2020047320 (print) | LCCN 2020047321 (ebook) |
ISBN 9780190066376 (paperback) | ISBN 9780190066390 (epub) |
ISBN 9780190066406
Subjects: MESH: Upper Extremity | Pain—diagnosis | Pain Management |
Case Reports
Classification: LCC RB127 (print) | LCC RB127 (ebook) | NLM WE 805 |
DDC 616/.0472—dc23
LC record available at https://lccn.loc.gov/2020047320
LC ebook record available at https://lccn.loc.gov/2020047321

DOI: 10.1093/med/9780190066376.001.0001

9 8 7 6 5 4 3 2 1

Printed by Marquis, Canada

Contents

Preface

This volume of the What Do I Do Now (WDIDN) Pain Medicine series presents clinical scenarios related to painful syndromes affecting the upper limb. Emphasis is placed on common presenting symptoms and diagnoses expanding into more complex conditions requiring extensive diagnostic evaluation and complex management strategies.

Upper limb pain can be challenging to evaluate and manage given the multiple etiologies, complex anatomical structures, and pain referral patterns. Syndromes affecting the upper limb can lead to significant disability affecting individuals in their daily life activities and their occupations. Common cumulative trauma disorders and their resulting functional and vocational effects will be discussed with special attention to rehabilitative management and functional restoration. The interplay of neuromusculoskeletal structures and function in the upper limb will be front and center pieces of the cases.

The chapters of this book were written by a group of authors with whom I have maintained professional and personal relationships over my career. Their training and expertise expand several medical specialties including Physical Medicine & Rehabilitation, Anesthesia/Pain Management, Orthopedic Surgery, Spine Surgery, and Hand Surgery. Their combined years of experience listening to countless patients and providing expert compassionate care are reflected throughout the book.

The authors have placed meticulous emphasis on proper diagnosis and management options for these syndromes using specific restorative approaches. This has never been of greater importance in light of the current nationwide opioid epidemic. This volume focuses on nonopioid and mostly nonpharmacological management methods for painful syndromes affecting the shoulder, arm, and hand. The discussions are highly relevant and useful for providers in primary care settings as well as specialty care. On behalf of all the authors and mine, we thank you for your interest in reading this book and sincerely hope you will find it useful to continue caring for patients with upper limb ailments.

Acknowledgments

I would like to thank all the authors for their phenomenal contributions to this book. Their combined expertise and passion have made this volume whole. Special thanks to all the residents and medical students that I have had the honor of teaching throughout my career. Sharing my knowledge has always been my Hippocratic duty and has undoubtedly challenged me to continue learning.

I would also like to thank the countless patients who have taught me about compassion and the unyielding resilience of the human spirit, along with the incredible complexities of the human body. And lastly, my heartfelt thanks to my wife María Claudia and my children Laura and Andrés for their unwavering support and patience during this project and my entire career.

Contributors

Mamun Al-Rashid, MD, MRCS, FRCS, FACS
Director Adult Reconstruction
    Surgery, Board Certified
    Orthopedic Surgeon
Department of Orthopedic
    Surgery
Atlantis Orthopedics
Associate Professor of Orthopedic
    Surgery
Larkin Orthopedic
    Residency, Miami
Affiliate Assistant Professor of
    Medical Education
University of Miami Miller School
    of Medicine
West Palm Beach, FL, USA

Caitlin M. Cicone, DO
Interventional Spine and
    Musculoskeletal Physiatrist
Department of Neuroscience Spine
    Center (PM&R)
Baptist Hospital South Florida
Miami, FL, USA

Ady M. Correa-Mendoza, MD
PM&R Service
VA Caribbean Healthcare
    System
San Juan, PR, USA

Maricarmen Cruz-Jimenez, MD
Associate Chief of Staff for
    Education
Physical Medicine and
    Rehabilitation Service
VA Caribbean Healthcare System
San Juan, PR, USA

Ramon Cuevas-Trisan, MD
Associate Chief of Staff for
    Education & Research
West Palm Beach VA Medical
    Center
Riviera Beach, FL

Melissa Guanche, MD
Interventional Spine Physiatrist
Miami Neuroscience Institute
Baptist Health
Miami, FL, USA

Anne-Sophie Lessard, MD, FRCSC, FACS
Assistant Professor of Surgery
Division of Plastic and
    Reconstructive Surgery
University of Miami Miller School
    of Medicine
Miami, FL, USA

Leland Lou, MD
Private Practitioner
Demopolis, AL, USA

Amir Mahajer, DO, FAOCPMR, FAAPMR, CAQSM
Interventional Physiatrist of Spine
  at Mount Sinai West
Department of Orthopedics and
  Sports Medicine
Assistant Professor of Orthopedic
  Surgery, Rehabilitation &
  Human Performance
Icahn School of Medicine at
  Mount Sinai
New York, NY, USA

Julio A. Martinez-Silvestrini, MD
Medical Director
Baystate Rehabilitation Care
Baystate Health
Westfield, MA, USA

John Melendez-Benabe, MD
Chief, Pain Management Section
Physical Medicine & Rehabilitation
  Service
Department of Veterans Affairs
  Medical Center
West Palm Beach, FL, USA

William J. Molinari, III, MD
Orthopedic Spine Surgeon
Department of Surgery
Department of Veterans Affairs
  Medical Center
West Palm Beach, FL, USA

Keryl Motta-Valencia, MD
Attending Physician
Physical Medicine and
  Rehabilitation Service
VA Caribbean Healthcare
  System
San Juan, PR, USA

Quynh Giao Pham, MD
Pain Medicine Fellowship Program
  Director
Department of Physical Medicine
  and Rehabilitation
VA Greater Los Angeles
  Healthcare System
West Los Angeles, CA, USA

Matthew Robinson, DO
Pain Medicine Fellow
Department of Physical Medicine
  and Rehabilitation
VA Greater Los Angeles
  Healthcare System
West Los Angeles, CA, USA

Sriram Sankaranarayanan, MD
Assistant Professor
Department of Orthopaedic
  Surgery
NYU School of Medicine
New York, NY, USA

Joyti Sharma, MD
Physician
Pain Management Section, Physical
    Medicine & Rehabilitation
    Service
Department of Veterans Affairs
    Medical Center
West Palm Beach, FL, USA

Amanda Spielman, BS
Medical Student
Division of Plastic, Aesthetic, and
    Reconstructive Surgery
University of Miami Miller School
    of Medicine
Miami, FL, USA

Bruno Subbarao, DO
Attending Physician
Physical Medicine and
    Rehabilitation Service
Phoenix Veterans
    Healthcare System
Phoenix, AZ, USA

1 Sandpaper Sensation in the Shoulder

Ramon Cuevas-Trisan

A 66-year-old right-handed male complains of progressive painful "grinding" in his right shoulder. He plays recreational tennis several times per week and these symptoms are affecting his game (serving has become extremely difficult and painful). He complains of morning stiffness and a "clicking" sensation with certain arm movements. He plays mostly doubles because his knees also bother him. Pain is generally minimal to absent when resting, and he denies any shortness of breath, palpitations, abdominal pain, neck pain, or tingling or numbness sensation in the arm. He has taken acetaminophen and ibuprofen, reporting minimal improvement. His past history is remarkable for high blood pressure, peptic ulcer disease, and benign prostatic hyperplasia. He underwent cholecystectomy and abdominal hernia repair years ago. Directed examination shows no gross deformity, mild limitation in active range of motion of the shoulder (mainly external rotation and abduction) with palpable crepitus, no tenderness, and impingement signs are negative. He has good distal strength, and sensation is normal.

What do you do now?

- Are this patient's symptoms related to intrinsic or extrinsic shoulder pain generators?
- If the pain is coming from intrinsic shoulder structures, is the problem at the glenohumeral joint or extraglenohumeral structures?
- What additional history details should you seek and what additional workup should you perform at this time?

Shoulder pain is a common musculoskeletal complaint that may be due to intrinsic shoulder structures or represent a referred pain pattern. The shoulder is a very complex anatomical structure with a tremendous degree of mobility in a multitude of directions, making it the joint with greatest mobility in the human body. The shoulder girdle has three bones (proximal humerus, clavicle, and scapula) and articular surfaces [glenohumeral (GH), acromioclavicular (AC), sternoclavicular, and scapulothoracic]. Its principal one, the GH joint, is very shallow and is mainly held in place by a complex array of soft tissues, allowing for a very large degree of mobility but making it susceptible to instability. The glenoid labrum in its outer rim is a fibrocartilaginous structure that provides an additional amount of depth to this ball-and-socket joint. Extrinsic stabilizers include static (GH ligaments and joint capsule) and dynamic (rotator cuff, teres major, latissimus dorsi, and pectoralis major) components. The rotator cuff is composed of four muscles: one primary abductor and external rotator (supraspinatus), two primary external rotators (infraspinatus and teres minor), and one primary internal rotator (subscapularis). The rotator cuff stabilizes the humoral head in the glenoid fossa, counterbalancing the elevating forces of the deltoid while maintaining contact between the humeral head and the glenoid fossa (normally only 25% surface contact). Weakness or mechanical deficiency of the rotator cuff can lead to superior subluxation of the humeral head when the shoulder is abducted, predisposing to impingement syndromes. The suprascapular nerve innervates the supraspinatus and infraspinatus muscles.

The complex kinematic interaction between the various shoulder joints is known as the scapulohumeral rhythm, which is a carefully coordinated ratio of movement among these joints to produce smooth arm elevation.

The evaluation of shoulder complaints is dictated first by the presence of trauma and potentially dangerous extrinsic causes of shoulder pain. These extrinsic causes are mainly evaluated during careful history taking, focusing on the individual's risk factors and pain pattern, particularly as related to any movement or activity because extrinsic causes generally display a pain pattern that is not specifically related to arm movements. Pain with these conditions also tends to be somewhat vague poorly localized and include referred pain due to diaphragmatic irritation (spleen/liver pathology or bleeding), acute coronary syndrome/angina, suprascapular nerve injury and referred pain from cervical spine pathology (radiculopathy/facet-generated pain/herpes zoster). Rarely, referred pain patterns from lung pathology (upper lobe pneumonia and apical lung tumor) may be seen. Patients with cervical spine pathology with pain radiating to the shoulder will usually show signs of neurological involvement, manifested by sensory (numbness or other sensory abnormalities such as paresthesias), motor (weakness), or muscle stretch reflex changes (hypo- or hyperreflexia). Common areas of sensory complaints involve the lateral shoulder, upper trapezius, scapular region, and the forearm and hand. In cases of trauma, it is important to rule out fractures (humerus, scapula, and clavicle), dislocations (GH and AC), or acute soft tissue injuries (traumatic rotator cuff tears, glenoid labrum tears, and nerve compression/stretch injuries). Box 1.1 summarizes shoulder pain etiologies systematically.

The time course of this patient's presentation along with the lack of trauma effectively rule out acute traumatic causes of shoulder pain. In this case, we would need to evaluate for intrinsic causes of shoulder pain focusing on distinguishing GH versus extra-GH causes of pain. Extra-GH causes mainly include tendinopathy/tear of the biceps tendon (most commonly the long head) and AC joint arthritis/sprain. The lack of tenderness and deformity (Popeye sign due to a tear of the long head of the biceps, scapular winging, or step deformity of the AC joint) does not support these diagnoses, pointing to possible GH causes. These include rotator cuff pathology (impingement, tear, and tendinopathy), adhesive capsulitis, labral tear, GH instability, and GH arthritis.

BOX 1.1   **Main Etiologies of Shoulder Pain**

Traumatic (Imaging Mandatory)

Fractures—clavicle, proximal humerus, scapula
Dislocations/sprain—GH, AC, SC

Extrinsic

Cervical—radiculopathy, zoster, zygoapophyseal joint arthropathy
Plexus and focal nerve lesions (i.e., suprascapular/axillary nerve palsy,
    thoracic outlet syndrome)
Visceral—diaphragmatic irritation (liver, spleen, gallbladder), cardiac

Intrinsic

Extraglenohumeral
    AC arthritis
    Scapulothoracic ailments
    Biceps tendonitis/tears
Glenohumeral
    GH instability
    Rotator cuff (tears, impingement, tendinopathy)
    GH arthritis (OA, osteonecrosis, crystal-induced, Rheumatoid
        Arthritis)
    Glenoid labrum tears
    Adhesive capsulitis

The limited information provided regarding this patient's clinical examination findings does not suggest rotator cuff pathology. Patients with rotator cuff damage often present with anterolateral shoulder pain, point tenderness, impingement signs (positive Neer and Hawkins tests), and other abnormalities on examination (drop arm test, specific painful arc, and positive empty can test). Adhesive capsulitis is more prevalent in diabetic individuals and tends to affect range of motion in all directions profoundly. It is also seen as a consequence of trauma (musculoskeletal or neurological), with a resulting immobilizing disability leading to disuse. The presence of arthritis, instability, or a labral tear cannot be fully excluded with the information provided. Labral tears can be seen acutely due to trauma or, more commonly, chronically as a result of repetitive injuries. This individual's recreational sports activities can certainly be a risk factor for cumulative trauma/injury. Further evaluation of this can be accomplished on physical examination by performing other tests (e.g., the O'Brien test) and searching for a clicking, catching, or locking sensation in cases of the most common type of labral tear, the superior labrum anterior to posterior lesion (SLAP), but generally requires performing magnetic resonance imaging (MRI). GH Instability is typically detected on physical examination by excessive passive displacement of the head of the humerus in the glenoid fossa in multiple directions. Patients with this condition may present with a "sulcus sign" deformity and often have a positive "apprehension test," the patient feels as if the shoulder is going to dislocate as the examiner passively manipulates it into abduction and external rotation. This is a common ailment in competitive swimmers, gymnasts, weightlifters, and some throwing athletes, generally as a result of cumulative stretching of the soft tissues over time.

In this patient, additional examination maneuvers did not reveal any clicking or locking, the O'Brien test was negative, and no instability, apprehension, or sulcus sign were detected. The limitations in range of motion were noted both passively and actively, toward the end of the range in abduction and external rotation. Sensation throughout the arms was normal, and strength and reflexes were symmetric and normal.

The examination findings along with the patient's history are highly suggestive of osteoarthritis (OA) of the GH joint. The patient had also complained of knee pain while playing tennis, also pointing to the possibility of a more widespread problem such as OA.

Osteoarthritis of the GH joint is seen as wear and tear of the articular cartilage of the glenoid, the glenoid labrum, and the head of the humerus. In the vast majority of cases, a history of prior trauma (either an episode sometimes many years prior, such as dislocation, humeral fractures, or rotator cuff tears, or repetitive/cumulative the years) is elicited. Pain generally presents in a gradually progressive manner over the course of months to years and tends to be described as a deep ache in the anterior shoulder that worsens with activities requiring use of the arm. Rare conditions that may lead to degenerative changes of the GH joint include atraumatic osteonecrosis (seen in the setting of corticosteroid therapy and significant ethanol consumption) and inflammatory conditions such as crystal-induced arthropathies and rheumatoid arthritis.

Plain shoulder radiographs were taken and are shown in Figure 1.1. These show significant degenerative changes of the GH joint as seen in moderate to severe OA (subchondral sclerosis, marginal osteophytes, flattening of the humeral head, and narrowing of the joint space). Given all the findings, the clinician correctly decided to not seek additional workup with an MRI.

When there is no history of trauma, an anteroposterior (AP) view may be sufficient. However, in cases of trauma, axillary and scapular "Y" views are warranted because these may reveal dislocation and fractures that can be missed on AP views alone.

MRI is the preferred imaging study for patients with suspected rotator cuff ailments or glenoid labrum pathology. It is also useful in the evaluation of avascular necrosis, biceps tendinopathy and rupture, inflammatory processes, and tumors. This imaging modality has largely replaced arthrography except in cases in which adhesive capsulitis is suspected.

Ultrasound is currently widely used. Its diagnostic accuracy in expert hands can be close to that of MRI in identifying some soft tissue pathologies. Injection tests can also be performed to yield additional information about pain-generating structures, particularly in cases in which multiple pathological processes are suspected. These injections can be both diagnostic and therapeutic (using local anesthetic alone or in combination with a steroid) and can focus on different structures, including the GH joint, the subacromial bursa, the tendon sheath of the long head of the biceps, or the AC joint. Ultrasound guidance has mostly become the standard when performing these injections to ensure accuracy of placement.

Management of this condition should proceed using a stepwise approach. Initial medical and conservative management can be achieved with physical therapy and basic analgesics, both oral topical. Physical therapy should focus on strengthening relatively weak muscles around the shoulder girdle in order to achieve balance and multidirectional stability of GH movements. It is common to see patients whose biceps and deltoid are strong and well developed their scapular stabilizers and small rotators are significantly weak. This often leads to repetitive microtrauma that results in premature degenerative joint changes. It is also common to see areas of muscle and soft tissue tightness that may cause undue restriction of certain joint movements. These should be addressed by a program involving gradual stretching. Self-application of cold and warm compresses as well as therapeutic electrical stimulation can help in the overall program.

Corticosteroid injections are often used. These are mostly used for short-term control of painful symptoms but do not alter the progression of the disease. Injection of hyaluronic acid compounds into the GH joint is not approved by the U.S. Food and Drug Administration but is done in the United States as well as other countries, where some of these commercially available products are approved for use in joints other than the knees. These injections can be done with ultrasound guidance or fluoroscopically. Other injectables, including platelet-rich plasma, mesenchymal stem cells, and "proliferant" agents (prolotherapy with hypertonic saline or highly concentrated glucose and others to induce inflammation and promote tissue repair), are used, but there is limited evidence regarding their efficacy.

Surgical options are generally considered when conservative care has not been successful. Joint preservation surgical approaches are generally considered in younger patients, generally those younger than 60 years. Some of these approaches include arthroscopic debridement, capsular release, synovectomy, and corrective osteotomies, all based on the patient's symptoms and limitations. Shoulder arthroplasty is the treatment of choice in cases of severe GH OA. Arthroplasty may involve the replacement of one or both components of the joint (glenoid socket and humeral head). Reverse arthroplasty (in which the "socket" component is replaced on the humeral head and the "ball" component is replaced on the glenoid socket) is used in cases of full rotator cuff tears and some cases of prior failed surgery. This type of implant makes the deltoid more efficient. Outcomes of shoulder arthroplasty are generally good, with total shoulder replacement typically yielding superior results compared to hemiarthroplasty. However, shoulder replacement surgery is still considered a treatment of last resort in cases of severe shoulder OA.

KEY POINTS TO REMEMBER

· The prevalence of shoulder OA is higher in whites, males older than 45 years and females older than 55 years, and overweight and inactive persons.

- When evaluating patients with shoulder pain, it is important to use a systematic approach, initially separating extrinsic (referred pain) and intrinsic (pain from the shoulder girdle structures) causes followed by evaluation of GH versus extra-GH causes or pain.
- Evaluation of shoulder pain in the setting of an acute traumatic injury mandates imaging studies, whereas in the setting of nontraumatic history, imaging requirements should be carefully guided by the patient's history and examination findings.
- Management of shoulder OA should follow a stepwise approach from conservative to minimally invasive and, last surgical.

Further Reading

Ansok CB, Muh SJ. Optimal management of glenohumeral osteoarthritis. *Orthop Res Rev*. 2018;10:9–18.

Khazzam M, Gee A, Pearl M. Management of glenohumeral joint osteoarthritis. *J Am Acad Ortho Surg*. 2020 (June 9):E-Pub ahead of print. doi:10.5435/JAAOS-D-20-00404

Macias-Hernandez SI, Morones-Alba JD, Miranda-Duarte A, et al. Glenohumeral osteoarthritis: Overview, therapy and rehabilitation. *Disab Rehabil*. 2017;39(16):1674–1682.

Millet PJ, Fritz EM, Frangiamore S, Sandeep M. Arthroscopic management of glenohumeral arthritis: A joint preservation approach. *J Am Acad Ortho Surg*. 2018;26(21):745–752.

Thomas M, Bitwai A, Rangan A, et al. Glenohumeral osteoarthritis. *Shoulder Elbow*. 2016;8(3):203–214.

2 A Softball Weekend Warrior's Nightmare

Julio A. Martinez-Silvestrini

A 45-year-old right-handed male without any known history of systemic illnesses is complaining of right shoulder pain for the past 3 months. His symptoms started approximately 1 month after his recreational softball season started. He describes pain localized to the lateral aspect of his right shoulder with certain arm movements. He denies any neck pain or numbness or tingling involving his right arm or hand. Nevertheless, he has an achy sensation on the lateral aspect of his arm, going down to below his deltoid. He is having difficulty buckling his seat belt, putting on a jacket, and sleeping on his right shoulder.

On physical examination, there is tenderness to palpation on the right subacromial space. There is no tenderness over the bicipital groove. He has essentially full shoulder range of motion but pain with abduction and with resisted external rotation and abduction. He has otherwise normal strength and no sensory loss. His muscle stretch reflexes are symmetric and normal.

What do you do now?

- Rotator cuff tendinopathy
- Rotator cuff tear
- Biceps tendonitis
- Adhesive capsulitis (frozen shoulder)
- Acromioclavicular osteoarthritis/sprain
- Cervical radiculopathy
- Brachial plexopathy

Shoulder impingement syndrome is the most common shoulder disorder, seen in 44–65% of patients complaining of shoulder pain. This syndrome may include multiple entities, such as subacromial bursitis, rotator cuff (RC) tendinopathy, and biceps tendinopathy. It is not uncommon for more than one of these conditions to occur at the same time. The patient's history and physical examination are most consistent with subacromial bursitis and RC tendinopathy (also known as tendonitis or tendinosis), involving both the supraspinatus and infraspinatus tendons. The diagnosis of subacromial bursitis is suspected when there is local tenderness to palpation on the area of the bursa (Figure 2.1). Patients with RC tendinopathy complain of lateral shoulder pain (Figure 2.1), but the diagnosis is made by pain with recruitment of the RC musculature. The RC complex is composed of four muscles: supraspinatus, infraspinatus, teres minor, and subscapularis. These four muscles can be easily recalled by the mnemonic SITS. The supraspinatus assists the deltoid with abduction of the shoulder, whereas the infraspinatus and teres minor are the main external rotators of the shoulder. The subscapularis assists the pectoralis muscle and latissimus dorsi with internal rotation of the shoulder. Disorders involving this "cuff" may occur traumatically, but most often they are secondary to chronic overload or overuse syndrome. This patient confirms that he had been participating in softball and after 1 month started experiencing his symptoms. He denies any acute trauma, which would be more concerning for a possible RC tear. It is important to keep in mind that in patients older than age 60 years, it is not uncommon to see calcific tendonitis (Figure 2.2) or RC tears that may occur without significant trauma.

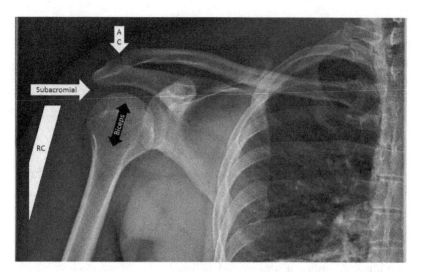

FIGURE 2.1 Right shoulder anteroposterior radiograph with common areas of tenderness according to diagnosis. AC, acromioclavicular joint; Biceps, biceps (long head) tendinopathy; RC, rotator cuff tendinopathy referred pain (usually not tender to touch); Subacromial, subacromial bursitis.

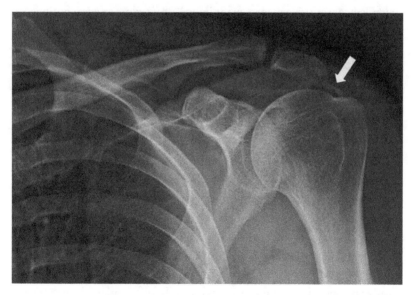

FIGURE 2.2 Left shoulder anteroposterior radiograph with evidence of calcific tendonitis (arrow).

This patient does not have tenderness over the bicipital groove (Figure 2.1), a finding commonly seen in patients with biceps tendinopathy. He has full range of motion and thus no evidence of adhesive capsulitis or frozen shoulder. Commonly, patients with adhesive capsulitis have significant limitation in range of motion with passive external rotation, which is a relatively pain-free maneuver that can be done in patients with shoulder pain. The patient does not complain of pain on the superior aspect of the shoulder and has no tenderness to palpation on the acromioclavicular (AC) joint (Figure 2.1), as commonly seen in patients with AC osteoarthritis or sprains. The patient has a normal peripheral neurological examination, with normal strength, sensation, and muscle stretch reflexes, for which the possibility of cervical radiculopathy will be less likely.

Because he persists with pain after 3 months, it is appropriate to obtain imaging studies to confirm that he has not developed calcifications in the tendon (calcific tendinopathy; Figure 2.1). Magnetic resonance imaging (MRI) is not recommended as the first imaging modality, particularly considering that the patient has normal strength and full active range of motion. MRI is considered if a tendon tear is suspected or when the patient has tried and failed conservative management in order to explore surgical options.

A high suspicion of an RC tear requires prompt, expeditious action. This should be suspected in patients with shoulder trauma or significant weakness. The RC musculature will atrophy, and there will be tendon fibers retraction approximately 4–6 months after injury. Therefore, after 6 months, surgical repair could become very difficult or impossible. If there is a suspicion of a RC tear in a relatively young and highly functional patient, an MRI should be obtained.

The presence of weakness, in combination with sensory loss or absent or decreased reflexes, may be indicative of a nerve injury. Nerve injuries that may mimic shoulder impingement include cervical radiculopathy and brachial plexopathy. Most patients with cervical radiculopathy have associated neck pain and pain with extension and lateral bending of the neck toward the affected side. An examination maneuver known as the Spurling test simulates this movement combination and is used as a provocative maneuver to test for that condition. To differentiate the presence of radiculopathy or plexopathy, an electrodiagnostic study (nerve conduction studies and electromyography) is recommended, usually after 3 weeks of the onset of symptoms. If this patient presented with hyperreflexia or spasticity, spinal pathology such as cervical spinal stenosis or myelopathy should be suspected and evaluated. In that case, cervical imaging would be recommended.

A good strategy for musculoskeletal care would be symptom control followed by rehabilitation. In the case of this patient, we are dealing with a young, very active, and otherwise healthy individual. Simple analgesics such as acetaminophen or nonsteroidal anti-inflammatory drugs (NSAIDs) can be considered for pain and reduction of inflammation. NSAIDs should be used carefully or may be contraindicated in geriatric patients and patients with significant cardiovascular disease, liver or kidney dysfunction, and a history of gastrointestinal ulcers or bleeding. In these patients, topical NSAIDs can be considered.

Once the patient's pain is better controlled, the rehabilitation program should focus on the patient's anatomic dysfunction (RC tendinopathy) and functional limitations (pain with certain shoulder/arm movements). Physical therapy modalities may include cold packs, superficial heat, deep heat (ultrasound), and electrical stimulation (including iontophoresis). This will help manage the patient's symptoms but may not provide long-term benefits. A directed rehabilitation program for long-term management of the condition should also include range-of-motion, strengthening, stretching, and postural exercises. Specific exercises aimed at strengthening the muscles of the rotator cuff should be considered to promote better biomechanics and glenohumeral stability.

Patients who have tried and failed conservative care can be considered for corticosteroid injections. Injections should not be the first line of care because the effects of injections alone without rehabilitation are short-lived, usually 1–3 months. The goal of injections is to decrease the patient's symptoms to attain a pain-free window to optimize the patient's rehabilitation potential. Other treatment options may include prolotherapy or injections of platelet-rich plasma.

If all of the previously mentioned measures fail and the patient persists with significant symptoms and dysfunction, MRI and surgical referral should be considered.

- Shoulder impingement syndrome is the most common cause of shoulder pain and is associated to pathology involving the subacromial bursa, RC tendons, and/or biceps tendon.
- RC and biceps tendinopathy are usually caused by arm overuse, although traumatic injuries may be seen.
- Imaging studies should be considered if the patient's symptoms persist after 2 or 3 months.
- MRI should be considered in patients with shoulder trauma and associated weakness or in patients with more chronic shoulder pain that has failed conservative management.
- Cervical imaging or electrodiagnostic studies should be considered in patients with neurologic findings, such as absent reflexes and/or sensory loss. Hyperreflexia or spasticity requires further evaluation with cervical imaging.
- Symptom control followed by rehabilitation are recommended for the management of shoulder impingement syndrome.
- Injections and surgical care are usually reserved for patients who have tried and failed conservative management.

Further Reading

Consigliere P, Haddo O, Levy O, Sforza G. Subacromial impingement syndrome: Management challenges. *Orthop Res Rev*. 2018;10:83–91.

Cook T, Lewis J. Rotator cuff-related shoulder pain: To inject or not to inject? *J Orthop Sports Phys Ther*. 2019;49(5):289–293.

Lewis J, McCreesh K, Roy JS, Ginn K. Rotator cuff tendinopathy: Navigating the diagnosis–management conundrum. *J Ortho Sports Phys Ther*. 2015;45(11):923–927.

Lin MT, Chiang CF, Wu CH, et al. Comparative effectiveness of injection therapies in rotator cuff tendinopathy: A systematic review, pairwise and network meta-analysis of randomized controlled trials. *Arch Phys Med Rehabil*. 2019;100(2):336–349.

Vandvik PO, Lähdeoja T, Ardern C, et al. Subacromial decompression surgery for adults with shoulder pain: A clinical practice guideline. *BMJ*. 2019;6(364):I294.

3 Achy Shoulder After Sunset

Maricarmen Cruz-Jimenez

A 54-year-old right-handed male reports right shoulder pain of approximately 3 months of evolution. He states that it started insidiously, and he does not recall any traumatic or precipitating event. Pain is in the anterior shoulder area. Initially it was mild and intermittent, but more recently it has gotten worse in intensity and nearly constant. This pain interferes with activities associated with overhead lifting and particularly with nighttime sleep. He has used nonsteroidal anti-inflammatory medications and had a shoulder injection at an urgent care clinic a few weeks ago. Both of these interventions only afforded minimal and short-lived relief.

On examination, there are no gross deformities or signs of inflammation noted over the patient's shoulder. Shoulders appear symmetric and well developed. Arm/hand sensation and strength appear normal except for some guarding and give-way weakness on shoulder flexion that appears to be due to pain. Active range of motion of the shoulder is normal with pain on flexion. There is no neck pain with normal active range in all planes. There is tenderness over the bicipital groove, and impingement tests are positive.

What do you do now?

- Is there an isolated soft-tissue injury of the shoulder, or is there a combination of structures that may be affected?
- Is it necessary to consider ordering some imaging studies in this case at this time? If so, what imaging tests should be considered?
- Do you suspect any neurological injury or pain referred from other structures (e.g., neck)?

This patient presents symptoms and examination findings consistent with a biceps tendinopathy. This condition's clinical etiologic spectrum includes inflammatory, degenerative, overuse-related, and traumatic. Tendonitis refers to a more acute event in which there is inflammation of the tenosynovium, in most cases involving the long head of the biceps tendon as it courses through the bicipital groove of the humerus. Although bicipital tendonitis can manifest as an isolated clinical complaint, it is more commonly seen associated with other shoulder pathologies, including rotator cuff disorders, impingement syndrome, glenoid labrum tears, bursitis, and acromioclavicular joint disorders. An isolated bicipital tendonitis may be seen in cases of trauma (direct or indirect), underlying inflammatory disease, and tendon instability. There is a continuum of the disease when symptoms persist unresolved, but the initial trigger is repetitive trauma and friction injury that results in sheer forces and inflammation of the tendon. Pathologies at the biceps (tendonitis, rupture, and instability in the form of subluxation and dislocation) predominantly affect its long head.

In contrast to tendonitis, the term biceps tendinopathy reflects the end of the clinical spectrum and refers to chronic degenerative problems, manifested as intratendinous changes and characterized by minimal inflammatory cells, disorganized collagen fibers, and neovascularization that lead to chronic pain and functional alterations. These structural changes predispose the tendon to recurrent microinjury and eventual tears.

The biceps has two heads. Its long head has an extra-articular and intra-articular origin distribution, arising from the supraglenoid tubercle of the scapula and the superior glenoid labrum within the capsule. The short head has an extra-articular origin at the apex of the coracoid process. The muscle inserts in a conjoined tendon at the tuberosity of the radius and the aponeurosis of the biceps brachii (Figures 3.1 and 3.2). The proximal part of the long head is vascularized by the ascending vessels of the anterior humeral circumflex artery; the distal biceps is vascularized by the branches of the brachial and deep brachial arteries. The hypovascular area of the tendon lies 1.2–3 cm from the proximal origin, at the groove territory. By crossing two joints, the shoulder and elbow, the biceps is involved in different motions: both shoulder and elbow flexion and supination of the forearm, its main and stronger movement. In addition, the biceps can assist shoulder abduction and adduction depending on the positioning of the humerus.

Tendons can repair after an acute injury. They first go through an inflammatory stage that lasts approximately 7 days. This stage is followed by a proliferative phase, which can last up to 21 days. This is followed by the remodeling stage, which can last from 3–6 weeks to 1 year. In chronic repetitive tendonitis, these phases become insufficient for timely remodeling of the tendon, resulting in degeneration and deterioration of the biomechanical properties of the tendon (tendinopathy). In this stage

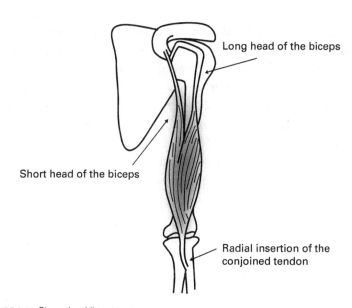

FIGURE 3.1 Biceps brachii anatomy.

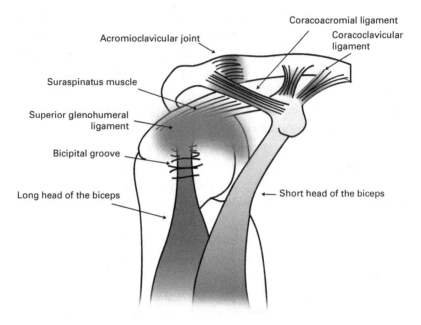

Coracoacromial ligament

Coracoclavicular ligament

Acromioclavicular joint

Suraspinatus muscle

Superior glenohumeral ligament

Bicipital groove

Long head of the biceps

Short head of the biceps

FIGURE 3.2 Schematic of the anatomical relationship between ligaments and tendons in the shoulder.

of injury, histologic studies show that inflammation is minimal or absent. Instead, myxoid degeneration and fibrosis are common findings. New disorganized growth of capillaries (neovascularization) is commonly seen, and spontaneous rupture becomes more probable. It is believed that this expansion of capillaries is accompanied by nerve endings, such as sensory and autonomic nerve fibers, that penetrate the tendons and become instrumental in the chronic pain cycle.

The intra-articular component of the long head of the biceps is susceptible to degeneration due to its frequent exposure to compression and friction forces. The extra-articular component is most commonly associated with the presence of rotator cuff tears.

The biceps tendon (long head) may be subject to subluxation or dislocation. When this happens, it is common to have concurrent rotator cuff pathology. In fact, medial subluxation of the long head of the biceps is a predictor for a subscapularis tendon tear.

Patients with bicipital tendonitis usually complain of dull and aching anterior shoulder pain. Many patients specifically localize the location over the bicipital groove. Instability is also a common symptom. When present, a history of previous trauma or dislocation is common. Depending on the chronicity and other accompanying causes, pain may extend throughout the muscle and include other neighboring structures, such as related bursae and rotator cuff tendons. Symptoms are of insidious presentation and may be accompanied by subacromial impingement complaints. Overhead activities tend to aggravate the pain.

Isolated bicipital tendonitis tends to occur in younger people who participate in tasks or sports that involve overhead activities (e.g., volleyball). When instability plays a role, patients often recall a specific event involving an audible "pop" or "click." Overhead and throwing activities may reproduce audible snaps. Subluxation of the tendon at the bicipital groove is most commonly attributed to subscapularis tendon partial or full tears. Tendinopathies of the biceps in older individuals tend to present more commonly as impingement of the shoulder and in combination with other structural pathology (e.g., rotator cuff).

Physical examination is very useful but has its limitations in establishing a clinical diagnosis for bicipital tendinopathy because other glenohumeral pathologies may present similar findings. In addition, the clinician should understand that shoulder examination maneuvers have varying degrees of sensitivity and specificity that can contribute to the clinical impression, and there is no specific combination of these that has a reliable positive predictive value for tendinopathy (Table 3.1). Due to sensitivity and specificity limitations of the clinical evaluation, the diagnostic workup will play an important role in confirming the diagnostic impression in bicipital tendonitis and tendinopathies. Workup can start with conventional plain radiographs of the shoulder. Although these are rarely helpful in establishing the diagnosis of bicipital tendonitis, they can exclude the presence of a primary generator for symptoms such as bone spurs, anatomic malformations, or other osteoarthritic changes. Magnetic resonance imaging (MRI) provides anatomical visualization of various pathological changes of the tendon, its location, and whether or not there is accumulation of fluid (edema). However, in biceps pathology, the MRI has been shown to have poor concordance with arthroscopic findings and poor to moderate sensitivity to

TABLE 3.1 **Useful Examination Findings for Biceps Pathology**

Examination Test	Method	Finding	Clinical Implication
Point tenderness	The tendon is palpated at the bicipital groove.	Focal tenderness	Tenosynovitis at the groove
Subpectoral tendon test	The tendon is palpated medial to the pectoralis major tendon insertion as the patient internally rotates the arm against resistance.	Focal tenderness	Tenosynovitis at the groove
Popeye sign	Observation	Gross deformity with distal retraction of the biceps muscle	Rupture of the long head of the biceps
Yergason test	The elbow is flexed at 90 degrees and stabilized against the thorax, at the same time the forearm is in pronation. The examiner resists supination of the forearm at the same time the arm is rotated laterally.	Positive test generates pain at the bicipital groove or the tendon may pop out of the groove.	Proximal biceps tendonitis
Speed test	The examiner resists shoulder forward flexion while the forearm is in supination and the elbow is in extension.	Positive test generates pain in the bicipital groove.	Tenosynovitis at the groove

TABLE 3.1 **Continued**

Examination Test	Method	Finding	Clinical Implication
O'Brien test	The shoulder is positioned in anterior flexion and 15 degrees of adduction. The patient is requested to resist downward pressure with the shoulder in maximal internal rotation and external rotation/supination.	Pain or painful clicking felt within the joint that improves with supination is a positive result.	SLAP lesion

SLAP, superior labral anterior posterior.

detect partial-thickness tears and ruptures. The sensitivity to detect partial or complete lesions of the long head of the biceps varies from 27% to 56%, respectively. When MRI is combined with arthrography, the sensitivity and specificity may increase, but differences are not significant. Arthrograms alone may show false-negative results in the presence of biceps pathology in 30% of cases.

Shoulder ultrasound is considered to have high accuracy in detecting normal biceps tendons and full-thickness tears but may not be as accurate in diagnosing partial-thickness tears or non-tear abnormalities such as tenosynovitis or tendinosis. Ultrasound has some diagnostic advantages, namely allowing functional evaluation of the structures, reproducing the pain by using provocative maneuvers that can identify specific sites of focal pain, and detection of tendon subluxations/dislocations. Arthroscopy, although invasive, remains the gold standard for the diagnosis of biceps tendinopathy.

Tendonitis of the biceps is initially managed conservatively, providing periods of relative rest and modification of provoking activities to allow healing and decreasing inflammation. Nonsteroidal anti-inflammatory drugs have a role in the early acute injury. Other modalities for pain management, including ice, heat, and topical ointments, can complement oral pharmacologic treatment. When these initial measures are unsuccessful, corticosteroid injections may help decrease inflammation of the tendon in its tenosynovial sheath and/or at its insertion. The initial attempt may include subacromial and glenohumeral joint injections. Medication injected to these spaces may spread to the biceps tendon sheath due to its continuity with the glenohumeral joint. Another approach is to inject the tendon sheath at the bicipital grove. This is commonly done using anatomical landmarks, but it is safer to perform under ultrasound guidance to avoid injecting the tendon and thus increasing the risk of rupture. Ultrasound-guided injections have a higher degree of accuracy compared with the blind (anatomical landmark) method.

Various regenerative therapies have also been described, including injection of platelet-rich plasma and proliferant therapy (prolotherapy) solutions. However, the evidence for their effectiveness is generally lacking. Regardless of the injectate, these injections are generally helpful, but correction of faulty biomechanics through proper exercises is essential for long-term recovery and secondary prevention. In this case, the patient received one such injection but no therapy afterwards.

Physical therapy has an important role in managing pain and the biomechanics of the shoulder, both in isolated bicipital tendonitis and when this is accompanied by other shoulder pathologies. In tendonitis of the biceps, and particularly when this is associated with other shoulder pathologies (e.g., rotator cuff tendinopathy), correcting faulty biomechanics of the shoulder is essential to rehabilitation and recovery. Among the rehabilitation considerations are correcting weakness of the affected muscles, correcting compensatory postures, and improving the scapular rhythm. These will lead to sustained long-term functional improvements. Another physical therapy modality, low-level laser therapy (LLLT), has been shown to be significantly superior in decreasing pain compared with placebo or no therapy, leading to significant analgesia. Pain improvements are also significantly better when laser is combined with exercise. Studies have shown that consistent effects are obtained when LLLT dosing follows the international recommended frequency guidelines of 780–904 nm. In chronic distal biceps tendinopathy, a single session of radial extracorporeal shock wave therapy has been shown to be a safe and effective way of reducing pain at 3 and 12 months.

Surgical intervention may be considered when conservative care has failed and there is persistent pain with functional limitations and in the presence of other shoulder pathologies. Indications for surgical management include partial-thickness tear of the long head of the biceps and medial subluxation of the long head, particularly if this is accompanied by a tear of the subscapularis tendon or the biceps pulley. Other indications for surgery include some types of superior labral anterior to posterior (SLAP) tears, chronic pain, and significant hypertrophy of the tendon.

Surgical management of pathology of the long head biceps tendon remains controversial, but two procedures have demonstrated effectiveness: tenotomy and tenodesis. Tenotomy involves partial slicing of the tendon to allow its lengthening. This procedure is preferred for being simple, has little postoperatory rehabilitation, and has predictable pain relief. Yet, its disadvantages are that cosmesis may be an issue and fatigue may occur. Up to 70% of cases may report a Popeye deformity, fatigue, and cramping with activities. Due to these problems, tenotomy is reserved for older patients, those who do not perform hard labor, and those who are not willing to go through lengthy postoperative rehabilitation. Tenodesis is the procedure that re-attaches a tendon to a bone. This procedure is performed when maintaining the length–tension relationship of the biceps muscle is the goal; this tension prevents postoperative atrophy and maintains the muscle contour. It is the preferred procedure in younger and active patients, athletes, manual laborers, and those who object to a potential muscle bulge/deformity above the elbow.

KEY POINTS TO REMEMBER

- Biceps tendinosis is a clinical spectrum that varies from acute tendonitis to chronic tendinopathy and full tears.
- The clinician should know that isolated tendonitis of the biceps is not common and that the biceps tends to dysfunction when other shoulder anatomical structures are injured. Understanding this concept will allow the clinician to focus on a comprehensive history and examination that will eventually lead to an accurate diagnosis and comprehensive rehabilitation plan.

- Initial conservative management should be considered in most patients except in younger/active individuals with full tendon tears where surgical correction may be undertaken.
- Injectable therapies, although usually helpful for reducing pain and inflammation initially, tend to provide only short-lived relief unless followed by physical therapy focusing on correction of biomechanical dysfunction.

Further Reading

Arnader M, Tennent D. Clinical assessment of the glenoid labrum. *Shoulder Elbow*. 2014;6(4):291–299.

Hashiuchi T, Sakurai G, Morimoto M, Komei T, Takakura Y, Tanaka Y. Accuracy of the biceps tendon sheath injection: Ultrasound-guided or unguided injection? A randomized controlled trial. *Shoulder Elbow Surg*. 2011;20(7):1068–1073.

Nho SJ, Strauss EJ, Lenart BA, Mazocca AD, Verma NN, Romeo AA. Long head of the biceps tendinopathy: Diagnosis and management. *J Am Acad Orthop Surg*. 2010;18(11):645–656.

Skendzel JG, Jacobson JA, Carpenter JE, Miller BS. Long head of biceps brachii tendon evaluation: Accuracy of preoperative ultrasound. *Am J Roentgenol*. 2011;197(4):942–948.

Streit JJ, Shishani Y, Rodgers M, Gobezie R. Tendinopathy of the long head of the biceps tendon: Histopathologic analysis of the extra-articular biceps tendon and tenosynovium. *Open Access J Sport Med*. 2015;6:63–70.

Varacallo M, Mair SD. Biceps tendon dislocation and instability. *StatPearls*. Treasure Island, FL: StatPearls Publishing. Retrieved September 7, 2019, from https://www.ncbi.nml.nih.gov/books/NBK534102

4 A Call to Thaw the Shoulder

Mamun Al-Rashid

A 55-year-old right-handed female presents
with a 4-week history of insidious pain in her
left shoulder (anterior and lateral). It is worse
at night, especially when she sleeps on her left
side. She started to notice her shoulder range
of motion deteriorating. She finds it difficult to
reach for overhead objects and has pain reaching
her seat belt when sitting in the front passenger
seat of vehicles. She denies any preceding
history of trauma or injury to the shoulder. Her
past medical history is significant for type 2
diabetes and recently diagnosed hypothyroidism.
She has had surgery for Dupuytren's disease of
her hands with good recovery.

On examination, she holds her arm by her side
in internal rotation. Active and passive range of
motion are severely limited in external rotation and
abduction. Pain is worse toward the end points of her
range and mostly located over the deltoid. Strength
is intact and symmetrical bilaterally. Neurological
examination is unremarkable.

What do you do now?

Several conditions can have overlapping symptomatology or concurrent presentations. These include glenohumeral osteoarthritis, calcific tendonitis, subacromial impingement syndromes, rotator cuff tendon tears, acromioclavicular joint osteoarthritis, adhesive capsulitis, and even unrecognized posterior shoulder dislocations. Other causes of referred pain to the shoulder, including degenerative cervical spine disease, must also be considered.

This patient's symptomatology and physical signs are highly suggestive of adhesive capsulitis (AC; also referred to as frozen shoulder) of the left shoulder. The insidious nature of her symptoms and the progressive global reduction in range of motion, particularly passive loss of external rotation and abduction, are the key components of the history and clinical examination. She also has significant risk factors in her past medical history, including diabetes, hypothyroidism, and Dupuytren's disease, which can predispose to the development of AC. It is also worth noting that AC can be provoked as a secondary event following prior trauma or surgery to the shoulder, mastectomy, and prior chest wall surgery, among others.

Other differential diagnoses must also be taken into account and excluded before proceeding with definitive treatment of this condition. AC is primarily a diagnosis made through a detailed history and careful physical examination. However, imaging studies can be a helpful adjunct in excluding other diagnoses and concurrent pathologies. Radiological studies include plain radiographs of the shoulder with a minimum of two views, such as anteroposterior and Y scapular views. These can be used to assess for acromioclavicular and glenohumeral osteoarthritis, subtle fractures, and calcifications in the subacromial space as well as subacute posterior dislocations of the humeral head. A magnetic resonance imaging (MRI) scan can help exclude concurrent conditions such as rotator cuff tears and superior labral anterior to posterior tears, and it may show thickening of the coracohumeral ligament and inferior glenohumeral joint capsule along with reduced dimensions of the rotator interval. MRI arthrography may show a volume reduction of the joint space.

Before initiating treatment, it is important to understand the pathophysiology and clinical stages of AC. The disease process is postulated to be a cytokine-induced synovial inflammatory process with fibrotic contracture of the rotator interval, glenohumeral capsule, and ligaments. Contracture of the coracohumeral ligament, which forms the roof of the rotator cuff interval, is thought to be the first structure/process involved, limiting external rotation. Subsequent thickening and contraction of the glenohumeral joint capsule limit further active and passive global range of motion of the shoulder joint.

Adhesive capsulitis is thought to progress through the following three clinical phases (stages) based on the timing of onset of symptoms: freezing, frozen, and thawing. However, it is important to note that these phases can overlap with concurrence of symptoms.

In the freezing phase (the first 2–9 months), the predominant symptom is diffuse pain around the shoulder. This is followed by the frozen phase (lasting 4–12 months), in which the pain can subside somewhat but there is progressive loss of global range of motion of the shoulder. Finally, during the thawing phase (lasting 5–26 months), there is a gradual recovery of the range of motion. For all practical purposes of management of this condition, it is important for the clinician to recognize the two stages of freezing and frozen. The typical course of AC from symptom initiation to self-limiting spontaneous resolution can span 1–3 years. However, certain early interventions can help avoid refractory persistence of this painful condition.

The mainstay of treatment of AC is nonsurgical treatment involving physical therapy with adjunctive pharmacotherapy. Pain management with nonsteroidal anti-inflammatory drugs (NSAIDs) and physical therapy should be part of the initial management. The timing of these interventions is critical because early intervention may prevent progression to severe stiffness and reduced range of motion of the shoulder. During the freezing phase, in which the shoulder is most painful, it is important to advocate for range-of-motion exercises within the pain tolerance range of the shoulder. These exercises include pendulum motion, passive supine forward elevation, external rotation, and active assisted range of motion in extension and horizontal adduction. Some studies have suggested that aggressive stretching beyond the pain threshold can result in poor outcomes, particularly in the early phase of the condition. Often, heat or cold packs can be applied as a modality to relieve pain before the start of these exercises. Additional adjunctive therapeutic ultrasound, cryotherapy, or transcutaneous electrical nerve stimulation may also be considered. Patients should be given a home exercise program to follow on a regular basis because this has demonstrated more success.

In the frozen phase, more aggressive stretching and range-of-motion exercises must be utilized to maintain and increase range of motion of the shoulder. In addition to stretching, strengthening exercises are added to maintain muscle strength.

Pain management is a key adjunct to allow patients to tolerate physical therapy and improve range of motion. NSAIDs may provide short-term pain relief. Oral corticosteroids have been used to improve disease treatment given the inflammatory nature of the early stages of AC. Several studies have shown, however, that the benefits of mainly pain relief are short-term and typically may not last beyond 6 weeks. Several studies have reported that intra-articular injection of methylprednisolone into the shoulder provided more rapid improvement in pain and range of motion. The benefit was sustained if complemented with physical therapy treatment. Others have reported that a series of one to three intra-articular injections of 40 mg of triamcinolone acetonide resulted in improved pain and shoulder disability scores compared to physical therapy alone for up to 1 year. Side effects of this treatment reported mainly in women include facial flushing and irregular menstrual bleeding. One additional option when pain limits progress in therapy is the use of suprascapular nerve or interscalene brachial plexus blocks to provide temporary pain relief in order to allow more effective physical therapy.

More invasive treatment options include manipulation under anesthesia (MUA) and arthroscopic capsular release. MUA may be considered in patients who have persistent pain and lack of improvement in range of motion despite 4–6 months of nonsurgical treatment. MUA produces a controlled stretching and tearing of adhesions under the joint capsule. The shoulder joint capsule is gently stretched by moving the humerus into flexion, abduction, and progressing to moving the adducted humerus into external rotation. However, there are some inherent risks to this procedure if not performed with due caution and gentle progression. Risks include soft tissue injuries to the shoulder such as labral tears, rotator cuff tears, hematomas, and even fracturing the humerus and joint dislocation. Arthroscopic capsular release involves controlled release of the soft tissues under direct visualization, specifically release of the rotator interval and anterior and inferior capsule. The posterior capsule can be selectively released when there is additional restriction of internal rotation. Many studies have demonstrated improvement in pain and range of motion of the shoulder, whereas others have reported recurrence rates of approximately 11% 1 year following the procedure. Certain subgroups of patients (patients with diabetes and those with postsurgical AC) have shown worse outcomes with the procedure.

KEY POINTS TO REMEMBER

- Adhesive capsulitis is a common shoulder condition that can be very painful and functionally disabling.
- Most cases are idiopathic, with a smaller number of individuals developing it secondary to previous trauma or surgery.
- The disorder has a predilection for middle-aged females, with risk factors including diabetes mellitus, thyroid disorders, and previous shoulder surgery.
- Adhesive capsulitis is a clinical diagnosis of painful shoulder with global loss of passive and active range of motion of the shoulder in the presence of normal radiological findings.
- Early diagnosis and intervention are important to achieve good outcomes.
- Initial treatment of AC should be nonsurgical with supervised physical therapy and self-directed exercises.
- Pharmacotherapy and steroid injections have demonstrated good short-term outcomes in improving pain control and shoulder function.
- Surgical treatment options should be reserved for patients with refractory symptoms in whom nonsurgical treatment has failed.
- Patient education regarding the natural course of the condition is very important to alleviate anxiety and frustration for the patient and enhance compliance.

Further Reading

Buchbinder R, Green S, Youd JM, Johnston RV. Oral steroids for adhesive capsulitis. *Cochrane Database Syst Rev.* 2006;2006(4):CD006189.

Bulgen DY, Binder AI, Hazleman BL, et al. Frozen shoulder: Prospective clinical study with an evaluation of three treatment regimens. *Ann Rheum Dis.* 1984;43:353–360.

Diercks RL, Stevens M. Gentle thawing of the frozen shoulder: A prospective study of supervised neglect versus intensive physical therapy in seventy-seven patients with frozen shoulder syndrome followed up for two years. *J Shoulder Elbow Surg.* 2004;13:499–502.

Van der Windt DA, Koes BW, Deville W, et al. Effectiveness of corticosteroid injections versus physiotherapy for treatment of painful stiff shoulder in primary care: Randomised trial. *BMJ.* 1998;317:1292–1296.

Watson L, Dalziel R, Story I. Frozen shoulder: A 12-month clinical outcome trial. *J Shoulder Elbow Surg.* 2000;9:16–22.

5 A Very Painful Arm with an "Alien" Inside

Ramon Cuevas-Trisan and Leland Lou

A 54-year-old female complains of diffuse pain and swelling of the left forearm and hand that started approximately 2 months ago and has gradually worsened. She denies any trauma. Her medical history is significant for generalized anxiety disorder, peptic ulcer disease, mild obesity, and prediabetes. Past surgical history includes a hysterectomy (4 years ago) and surgery for release of a left middle trigger finger 3 months ago. Pain is described as a deep ache and burning involving the "whole arm."

The dorsum of her hand is edematous, and the hand and forearm appear slightly erythematous. The left hand feels warmer to the touch compared with the right hand, and she is very guarded when you attempt to touch her hand. Any movement of the wrist is painful. There is a well-healed surgical scar in the palm of her hand without any overt signs of infection.

What do you do now?

The clinical presentation of this patient is very concerning. The degree of pain and symptoms appear to be limiting the use of her arm to a degree that could eventually lead to significant disability. Her relatively recent hand surgical procedure, although minor, raises concerns about potential infection/cellulitis or the presence of complex regional pain syndrome (CRPS). The description of a well-healed surgical scar and being afebrile lower the possibility of delayed surgical infection and cellulitis. The distribution of her symptoms (only one arm but not circumscribed to one joint) lowers the chances of this being an arthritic flare, as does the fact that there is no history of such chronic disorder. CRPS should be at the top of the diagnostic possibilities.

Complex regional pain syndrome mainly affects the extremities (arms/hands, legs/feet) but may affect any part of the body. It is often diagnosed in its chronic stages when there are significant functional impairments and disability. Symptoms may appear spontaneously but often follow some trauma or injury (including surgery). The preceding injury can be a fracture. Sprains and elective surgeries in the painful limb are also commonly described. Individuals without a history of injury should be carefully examined to ensure that another treatable diagnosis is not missed.

A hallmark of CRPS is continuous pain of high intensity, along with mild or dramatic changes in skin color, temperature, and/or edema in the affected area. CRPS is believed to be caused by damage to, or malfunction of, the peripheral and central nervous systems.

There are two types of CRPS: type I (formerly known as reflex sympathetic dystrophy, Sudek's atrophy, shoulder–hand syndrome, or algoneurodystrophy) and type II (formerly referred to as causalgia). Type II has an associated peripheral nerve injury, whereas type I does not. However, the validity of the two different forms continues to be investigated because some research has identified evidence of nerve injury in some type I patients.

The syndrome affects all ages and does not show any clear demographic distribution other than predominantly affecting females more frequently than males and average age at diagnosis from the late 40s to the early 50s. Studies of the incidence and prevalence of the disease show that many cases are mild and individuals recover gradually with time. In more severe cases, individuals may not recover and may develop long-term disability. Type I is the most common of the two types, and the medical literature often refers to this type when describing the syndrome.

Early diagnostic criteria were adopted by the International Association for the Study of Pain in 1994, but they have been replaced by the Budapest criteria described in 2003. Box 5.1 presents these criteria. It is important to note that these criteria include an element of disproportionality (pain that appears excessive to any injury) and being a diagnosis of exclusion (no other diagnosis that can explain the symptoms and signs).

Patients suffering from this syndrome are sometimes classified into two groups based on the temperature of the affected area. Patients are classified as having warm or hot CRPS (majority of patients) generally in the acute stages because this is a common vasomotor pattern early in its development. Patients classified as having cold CRPS are those seen in the more chronic stages. These patients have a higher prevalence of dystonias and tend to have a less favorable prognosis with a higher chance of chronic disability.

There are no specific tests for its diagnosis. It is a clinical diagnosis that sometimes is supported by some ancillary tests, including plain radiographs, triple-phase bone scans, thermography, electrodiagnostic tests, and sympathetic blocks. Testing is often necessary to help rule out other conditions, such as arthritic syndromes, Lyme disease, deep vein thrombosis, or polyneuropathies (e.g., from diabetes), because these require different treatment.

The use of imaging techniques is based on the observation that the disorder is often associated with excess bone resorption, resulting in patchy osteopenia/osteoporosis (sometimes referred to as post-traumatic osteoporosis). This is attributed to disuse of the limb (protective guarding) and can

BOX 5.1   **Budapest CRPS Clinical Diagnostic Criteria**

- Continuous pain, which is disproportionate to any inciting event
- At least one symptom in three of the following four categories:
  Sensory: Reports of hyperesthesia and/or allodynia
  Vasomotor: Reports of temperature asymmetry and/or skin color changes and/or skin color asymmetry
  Sudomotor/edema: Reports of edema and/or sweating changes and/or sweating asymmetry
  Motor/trophic: Reports of decreased range of motion and/or motor dysfunction (weakness, tremor, dystonia) and/or trophic changes (hair, nail, skin)
- Must display at least one sign at time of evaluation in two or more of the following categories:
  Sensory: Evidence of hyperalgesia (to pinprick) and/or allodynia (to light touch and/or temperature sensation and/or deep somatic pressure and/or joint movement)
  Vasomotor: Evidence of temperature asymmetry (>1°C) and/or skin color changes and/or asymmetry
  Sudomotor/edema: Evidence of edema and/or sweating changes and/or sweating asymmetry
  Motor/trophic: Evidence of decreased range of motion and/or motor dysfunction (weakness, tremor, dystonia) and/or trophic changes (hair, nail, skin)
- There is no other diagnosis that better explains the signs and symptoms

sometimes be detected by plain radiographs in the subacute/chronic stage. Bone scans can detect these changes sooner by showing a specific pattern of increased activity in the affected areas, namely increased blood flow, blood pooling, and delayed metabolism in the affected limb. However, reliance on a bone scan for the diagnosis of CRPS is controversial due to the variability of findings in many published studies. Bone densitometry has also been used for this purpose, but abnormal findings are variable and usually require a considerable amount of time to develop.

Electrodiagnostic testing (electromyography and nerve conduction studies) is often used because it provides one of the most accurate and reliable methods to diagnose injuries to the peripheral nerves. As such, these tests can be very beneficial in establishing an underlying nerve injury, the basic criteria to distinguish between CRPS type I and type II. These tests can also be crucial in determining that other conditions are not present to explain the patient's symptoms and signs. One challenging issue with these studies is the fact that many patients with allodynia and hyperalgesia are unable to tolerate them because testing tends to be uncomfortable even in asymptomatic patients.

Thermography is a method sometimes described as helpful in supporting the diagnosis of CRPS. This is based on the observation that in some cases, altered blood flow throughout an affected region may be measured. However, many other factors are known to contribute to altered thermographic readings (history of smoking, use of certain skin lotions, recent physical activity, and prior history of trauma to the region), and not all CRPS patients present with "vasomotor instability" (particularly in the later stages).

The patient in this case has a history of recent hand surgery. This was a rather minor and simple surgical procedure. Unfortunately, this event has led to a continuous pain state, which is disproportionate to the inciting surgery. She is clearly describing hyperesthesia/allodynia, warmth, changes in skin color, and swelling (Figure 5.1). Her range of motion is markedly decreased. All of these are essentially confirmed on physical examination, and there is probably no other diagnosis that better explains the signs and symptoms. In order to reach the latter conclusion, some diagnostic tests would be performed. In addition, a Doppler ultrasound to rule out a deep

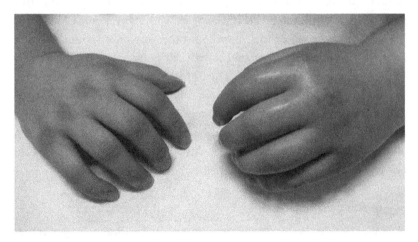

FIGURE 5.1 Physical appearance of the dorsum of the left hand compared to the asymptomatic hand.

vein thrombosis and a complete blood count to search for an infectious process are recommended.

MANAGEMENT METHODS

Delays in diagnosis and treatment of this syndrome can lead to severe physical and psychological problems. Early recognition and prompt treatment provide the greatest opportunity for recovery. Pain control in CRPS allows active participation in a rehabilitation regimen in order to restore motion and strength to the affected limb. Treatment for this condition is more successful when multiple modalities are combined, including educational, pharmacological, physical, interventional, and psychological, as outlined in the following sections.

Pharmacological Treatment

Pharmacological treatment is often one of the first lines of treatment. On the one hand, the least amount of medication needed tends to yield the best long-term results. On the other hand, to have any significant effect on controlling CRPS symptoms, a combination of medication classes may need to be used to address the various symptoms observed during the evolution of the disease. The key to success is to use analgesics to control pain in order for the patient to tolerate active exercises in therapy, always balancing efficacy with safety. Pharmacological and interventional modalities for pain control are used in a stepwise manner, beginning with those that are relatively safe and progressing to more risky interventions if a desired response is not initially achieved. There are no high-quality or comparative studies regarding efficacy for any individual drug or class of drugs in CRPS. Therefore, pharmacologic therapy is individualized based on the patient's age, comorbidities, concurrent medications, drug interactions, and side effects. For patients with early CRPS, this approach generally encompasses one or more of the agents discussed next.

Antiepileptic Medications

This medication group is a mainstay in all neuropathic pain syndromes despite limited data regarding efficacy. Although the pathogenesis of

CRPS is not well established, neurogenic inflammation and changes in central pain perception have been suspected to play a role, thereby providing rationale for use of medications with some evidence of benefit in other neuropathic pain conditions. Some of the most commonly used medications are the gabapentinoids, most commonly gabapentin. Carbamazepine and similar drugs have been used in the past, but their side effects profile has limited their use over time. Pregabalin is growing in use due to its increased bioavailability compared to gabapentin. Recently, gabapentinoids have been used more cautiously due to the growing awareness of the potential for misuse and abuse of these drugs as well as risk of respiratory dysfunction when used in combination with other central nervous system depressants.

Antidepressants

Depression is a common comorbidity in many patients with chronic pain syndromes. Antidepressants are commonly used as adjuvants in many neuropathic pain disorders and can also serve the purpose of addressing clinical depression when appropriately dosed. Tricyclic antidepressants such as amitriptyline, nortriptyline, and imipramine are used for neuropathic pain syndromes and often tried in CRPS in sub-antidepressant doses. Amitriptyline is frequently used for the additional benefit of addressing pain-related insomnia. A typical starting dose of amitriptyline or nortriptyline can be used (10–25 mg at bedtime or earlier in the evening if morning drowsiness occurs), followed by gradual increase in the dose, as tolerated. Several serotonin norepinephrine reuptake inhibitors (SNRIs) and selective SNRIs (e.g., venlafaxine, milnacipran, and duloxetine) have been used as well, with variable degrees of success.

Muscle Relaxants

Baclofen and tizanidine are common choices for muscle spasms in CRPS. Baclofen is thought to induce its effect by inhibiting the γ-aminobutyric acid B receptor and inhibiting both monosynaptic and polysynaptic reflexes at the spinal level. Tizanidine works via a central adrenergic α_2-agonist effect. The benzodiazepines can be effective as a muscle relaxant but should be used with caution due to their addictive potential.

Traditional Analgesics

Nonsteroidal anti-inflammatory drugs (NSAIDs) can help with analgesia and management of inflammation in CRPS. NSAIDs are well-known analgesics with no addictive potential. However, long-term use caries significant systemic risks, and these agents may need to be stopped when interventional procedures are included in the treatment plan due to the potential for bleeding complications.

Topical application of lidocaine (2–5%) and capsaicin (0.025–0.075%) cream is commonly used to treat neuropathic pain, but only limited data suggest efficacy in CRPS. These agents are probably best suited for patients with early CRPS and mild to moderate pain despite the use of anticonvulsants, antidepressants, and/or NSAIDs. They may be discontinued if they cause significant irritation or if there is no clinical benefit after a few days of use.

Opioids are efficacious for noxious pain treatment but are not the ideal first-choice pain medication. Whenever used, it must be with caution and always weighing the benefits versus the risks for a particular patient. Short-term use is generally not considered problematic, but long-term use has been associated with the potential for addiction.

Other Pharmacological Agents

Bisphosphonates have been used for the reduction of pain in CPRS patients with abnormal uptake on bone scan, based on evidence from several small randomized trials. The mechanism of analgesic effect in CRPS is unknown but is unlikely to be related to the antiresorptive properties of bisphosphonates. Proposed mechanisms include decreased proton concentration in the bone microenvironment, altering pain signal transduction via acid-sensitive ion channels, and decreased production of pro-inflammatory mediators such as tumor necrosis factor. Adverse effects of bisphosphonates are uncommon but may be serious, including esophageal ulceration with oral use and osteonecrosis of the jaw. Calcitonin has been used in some published studies that have produced weak evidence with the rationale of delaying bone resorption.

Oral glucocorticoids (divided doses of prednisone, 30–80 mg/day) have been studied for early stage CRPS, but there is only low-quality evidence from small randomized trials with substantial methodologic limitations. Findings from at least one small trial suggested that oral glucocorticoids are more effective than NSAIDs, but the risk of side effects and long-term toxicities outweighs potential benefits in most cases.

α-Adrenergic antagonists and agonists are sometimes used to address the sympathetically maintained pain believed to be part of the constellation of symptoms in some CRPS patients. Ketamine infusions are not uncommonly used in chronic and refractory CRPS cases, but systematic reviews have found that there is only low- to moderate-quality evidence supporting their use.

Nonpharmacological Modalities
Physical and occupational therapy are typically considered the mainstay first-line treatments for CRPS in order to prevent or quickly address functional impairments (range of motion limitations and prevention of contractures). These should be initiated as quickly as possible following a diagnosis of CRPS.

A variety of techniques can be used by therapists to address the symptom complex of CRPS. These include hydrotherapy, techniques for edema control, graded motor imagery, tactile and thermal desensitization (to normalize touch perception), mirror visual feedback, and stress loading. There is no definitive evidence in favor of any of these methods, but graded motor imagery may have the strongest evidence for reductions in pain and swelling in patients with CRPS in at least three small randomized clinical trials. Desensitization therapy is commonly used and may be assisted by topical medications such as lidocaine. In the authors' experience, other compounded topical creams may provide additional relief in select cases. Therapy must include range-of-motion and strengthening exercises to prevent adhesive capsulitis, soft-tissue contractures, maintain muscle mass, and reduce swelling. In some cases of CRPS, resting splints are used in order to prevent joint contractures. However, the effectiveness of splinting is uncertain and may in fact be detrimental. It is generally believed that early mobilization after limb injury/surgery may also reduce the risk of CRPS. For instance, patients with fractures require accurate assessment of fracture healing to strike an appropriate balance between proper fracture healing by immobilization and prolonged immobilization.

Ultimately, patients must learn ways to self-manage the condition on a daily basis. Patient participation in exercise regimens may be facilitated by clear explanation of the condition, including education about pain associated with CRPS, which is presumably related to neuropathic and central mechanisms but does not indicate tissue damage.

Interventional Pain Management Procedures

When patients do not improve with noninvasive therapy, interventional procedures may be considered. These may include trigger/tender point injections, sympathetic nerve blocks, spinal cord (dorsal column or dorsal root ganglia) stimulation, epidural clonidine, and chemical or mechanical sympathectomy.

There is very limited published high-quality evidence for these methods. However, in the authors' clinical experience, a number of patients derive meaningful benefit from these, when combined by progressive mobilization.

In the early stages of the condition, sympathetic nerve blocks may be highly beneficial, with edema reduction and improvement in normal blood flow to the affected limb. This is clinically apparent by increased temperature of the affected limb (if cool) and/or decreased pain. These procedures involve infiltration of a local anesthetic into the region of the relevant sympathetic ganglia (stellate ganglion for CRPS of the upper limb and lumbar sympathetic ganglion for CRPS of the lower limb), under fluoroscopic or ultrasound guidance. An alternative method for achieving sympathetic blockade is the slow intravenous injection of an anti-adrenergic drug such as guanethidine into the vein of the affected limb with a tourniquet applied to the extremity to occlude circulation (Bier block).

Intravenous local anesthetic infusions (i.e., lidocaine) have been used, but there are few supportive studies. Regional nerve blockage can be used as an acute treatment, but long-duration infusions can lead to significant complications including infections.

Peripheral nerve and/or spinal cord stimulation can be helpful in chronic CRPS management to treat the small and large nerve fiber changes. Spinal cord stimulation (SCS) is an invasive neuromodulation strategy that may be helpful if traditional therapeutic modalities fail, particularly in patients with disease limited to one extremity. A newer technique, dorsal root ganglia stimulation, has been used as the first choice of neuromodulation or in cases in which SCS has failed, with limited and emerging data suggesting superiority to traditional SCS and similar risks. Epidural clonidine administered via single injection or infusion may reduce pain in CRPS, but side effects such as hypotension and sedation are common.

Sympathectomy (chemical or surgical) is rarely used for CRPS due to its low-quality observational evidence and high rates of adverse effects, including increased pain, new neuropathic pain, and sweating abnormalities.

Psychological Assessment and Management

Psychological assessment and management, including cognitive–behavioral therapy, can be particularly effective in CRPS patients with preexisting or suspected psychologic or psychiatric issues and those who have insufficient improvement with the aforementioned treatment modalities. The goals are to identify any psychologic factors contributing to pain and disability, treat anxiety and depression, and provide the individual with effective coping strategies. Biofeedback therapy and guided imagery are commonly used techniques to control the autonomic dysfunction in CRPS.

KEY POINTS TO REMEMBER

- CRPS requires a multidisciplinary approach for successful management, including a combination of physical/occupational therapy, patient education, pharmacological management, and, in some cases, interventional procedures. Psychologic or psychiatric interventions may be needed in selected cases.
- Pharmacologic management and interventional procedures are used on an as-needed, individualized basis and using a stepwise approach. The main goal of these therapies is to provide some degree of analgesia that will allow the patient to tolerate graded activity and mobilization of the affected limb.
- Pharmacologic management may include NSAIDs, adjuvants (specifically anticonvulsants, antidepressants, and bisphosphonates), topical analgesics, α-adrenergic antagonists, and corticosteroids.

- Interventional pain management procedures used when managing CRPS should always be accompanied by progressive mobilization exercises.
- The prognosis of CRPS is quite variable, but many patients develop long-term dysfunction in the affected limb and long-term disability.

Further Reading

Atkinson L, Vile A. Unravelling the complex regional pain syndrome enigma. *Pain Med.* 2020;21(2):225–229. https://doi.org/10.1093/pm/pnz150

Birklein F, Dimova V. Complex regional pain syndrome-up-to-date. *Pain Rep.* 2017;2(6):e624. doi:10.1097/PR9.0000000000000624

Goh EL, Chidambaram S, Ma D. Complex regional pain syndrome: A recent update. *Burns Trauma.* 2017;5:s41038–016–0066–4. https://doi.org/10.1186/s41038-016-0066-4

Harden RN, Bruehl S, Stanton-Hicks M, Wilson PR. Proposed new diagnostic criteria for complex regional pain syndrome. *Pain Med.* 2007;8(4):326–331. https://doi.org/10.1111/j.1526-4637.2006.00169.x

National Institute of Neurological Disorders and Stroke. Complex regional pain syndrome fact sheet. Retrieved September 20, 2020, from https://www.ninds.nih.gov/Disorders/Patient-Caregiver-Education/Fact-Sheets/Complex-Regional-Pain-Syndrome-Fact-Sheet

Popkirov S, Hoeritzauer I, Colvin L, et al. Complex regional pain syndrome and functional neurological disorders—Time for reconciliation. *J Neurol Neurosurg Psychiatry.* 2019;90:608–614.

6 A "Spooky" Shoulder Blade

Joyti Sharma and

John Melendez-Benabe

A 22-year-old right-handed male tennis player presents with right shoulder pain, weakness, and instability. He reports ongoing symptoms for the past 3 months, including achy pain along the base of his neck, over the scapula, and over the deltoid region. He also reports having shoulder weakness and restricted range of motion.

Inspection shows slight winging of the right scapula, further accentuated when he is asked to forward flex his arms to horizontal and push up against the wall. No muscle atrophy is noted. There is mild tenderness to palpation along the upper and middle trapezius on the right. Taut bands are also present along the right medial border of the scapula.

Range of motion of the right shoulder is restricted (flexion and abduction to 120 degrees). Muscle strength is normal throughout the arms. Cranial nerves II–XII are intact. Sensation is grossly intact throughout both arms. Provocative maneuvers (Spurling's and Hawkins Tesys) are negative bilaterally.

What do you do now?

- Scapular winging (various types)
- SICK scapula
- Rotator cuff disorders
- Glenohumeral instability
- Peripheral nerve disorders
- Cervical spine disorders (e.g., cervical spondylosis, radiculopathy)
- Thoracic outlet syndrome
- Superior labral anterior to posterior lesion
- Bicep tendonitis
- Brachial plexopathy
- Scapular osteochondroma

The evaluation of a patient with shoulder dysfunction should always involve inspection of the scapula to screen for scapular winging. There may be abnormalities in static/resting position or its dynamic function characterized by medial border prominence or superior/inferior angle lateral displacement. This can affect the ability to abduct, flex, lift, and push. When clear scapular winging is observed, evaluation should focus on addressing possible causes of it. Scapular winging is a relatively uncommon problem that can often present with symptoms commonly seen in other shoulder and neck disorders. Diagnosis is usually achieved by a careful history and clinical examination including certain provocative maneuvers. Additional diagnostic testing, specifically using electrodiagnostic tests, can provide further assistance in determining the underlying neuromuscular pathology (i.e., damage to the long thoracic and spinal accessory nerve) as well as rule out other etiologies such as cervical radiculopathy or brachial plexopathy. The benefit of these measures is that early diagnosis and treatment can help prevent more severe shoulder dysfunction and unnecessary or unsuccessful surgical procedures.

Plain x-rays of the neck, chest, shoulder, and thoracic inlet are rarely diagnostic, but they should be obtained to rule out other structural abnormalities. Computed tomography and magnetic resonant imaging are rarely needed but may be useful to help rule out other diagnoses, such as disc pathology/radiculopathy and mass lesions.

Based on this patient's presentation, the most likely cause of the symptoms is a lesion to the long thoracic nerve causing medial scapular winging due to serratus anterior weakness and other associated abnormalities. Scapular winging is a rare, painful, and debilitating condition that leads to limited functional abilities of the upper limb. This condition can be due to multiple etiologies, including lesions to the long thoracic nerve (serratus anterior weakness) and spinal accessory nerve (trapezius weakness). Rarely, it may also be due to lesions involving the dorsal scapular nerve that innervates the rhomboid muscles.

The most common cause of scapular winging is damage to the long thoracic nerve. This can be traumatic, nontraumatic, or idiopathic. Long thoracic nerve damage should be considered in a patient with a history of repetitive overhead movements who presents with scapular dyskinesis and the corresponding restriction of overhead arm motions. Dyskinesis occurs when the movement of the scapula relative to the thorax does not occur in a harmonious way, leading to overload of the glenohumeral joint and the various muscle groups involved, causing pain and restriction of movement. It has been documented in the literature that injury to the long thoracic nerve in the majority of cases is due to trauma. This trauma ranges from acute trauma with rapid onset of scapular winging to the more common scenario of presumed cumulative trauma from activities including repetitive occupational tasks (e.g., tasks performed by car mechanics, scaffolders, welders, carpenters, and laborers) and various sports (baseball, basketball, body building/weight lifting, bowling, football, golf, gymnastics, hockey, soccer, tennis, and wrestling).

The main function of the serratus anterior is to protract and rotate the scapula, keeping it closely opposed to the thoracic wall and optimizing the position of the glenoid for maximum efficiency during upper limb motion. A typical patient with this condition may present with pain around the affected shoulder that either arises spontaneously or is linked to some traumatic event.

Pain in the shoulder is usually localized over the region of the rhomboids and levator scapulae muscles due to spasm. Patients may also complain of shoulder weakness, and athletes may complain of reduced performance.

Upon physical examination, the classic medial scapular winging is usually evident at rest, with the medial and inferior border closer to the spine and lifted superiorly compared to the normal side. Scapular winging can be accentuated when the patient is asked to forward flex the arms to horizontal and/or push on a wall in a push-up motion. In this position, the vertebral border (medial) of the scapula lifts further from the thoracic wall due to loss of the serratus anterior scapular protraction (Figure 6.1). Scapular assessment may reveal a SICK scapula (*s*capular malposition, *i*nferior medial border prominence, *c*oracoid pain and malposition, and dys*k*inesis of scapular movement).

Injury to the spinal accessory nerve produces weakness of the trapezius muscle. The most common cause for this type of injury is iatrogenic, generally after cervical lymph node biopsies and similar surgical interventions. The resulting scapular abnormality is often referred to as lateral scapular winging. A typical patient with this condition may present with stiffness, pain, and weakness of the shoulder girdle, especially with overhead activity

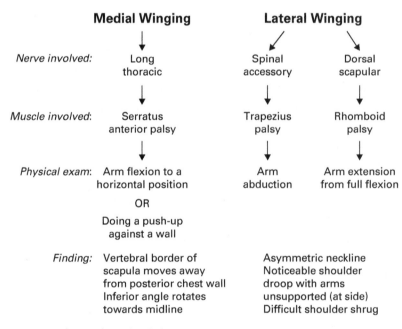

FIGURE 6.1 Causes of scapular winging.

and upon prolonged exertion. Pain can be quite debilitating, and patients may complain of a dull ache and heaviness around the shoulder, limiting overhead activities.

Physical examination reveals an asymmetric neckline with dropping of the affected shoulder. This may be accompanied by lateral displacement (winging) of the scapula. Typically, winging is minimal and accentuated during arm abduction. Winging may disappear during forward flexion of the arm due to the action of the serratus anterior muscle. Difficulty with abducting the arm is a consistent finding. The patient can also externally rotate the shoulder against manual resistance. Most cases of lateral winging of the scapula are due to spinal accessory nerve palsy (Figure 6.2).

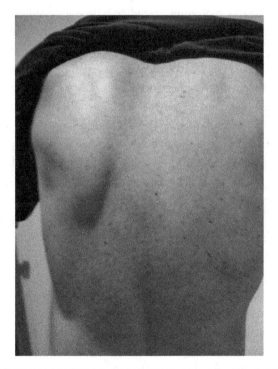

FIGURE 6.2   Medial scapular winging due to long thoracic nerve palsy. Note that the patient's left scapula is displaced away from the thoracic wall, and the inferior angle is slightly rotated toward the midline.

Courtesy of Dr. Ramon Cuevas-Trisan.

Injury to the dorsal scapular nerve will affect the function of the rhomboid muscles. A typical patient with this condition will present with pain down the medial aspect of the scapula, with pain sometimes radiating down the arm to the C5 and C6 dermatomes. The patient may also have a feeling of abnormal shoulder motion or traction when raising the affected arm. It generally produces very subtle winging of the scapula, with the scapula laterally translated and inferior angle rotated laterally. Winging could be accentuated by having the patient extend their arm from a fully flexed position. Due to the rhomboid anatomical position deep to the trapezius muscle and subtleness of the scapular winging, rhomboid paralysis is difficult to detect by clinical examination.

Many patients suffering from scapular winging eventually recover most or all functionality with proper management. However, if left untreated, several consequences can ensue, including adhesive capsulitis, subacromial impingement, and brachial plexus traction injuries. The recommended treatment for scapular winging associated with serratus anterior palsy is usually conservative. This can include physical therapy, pain management with analgesic or anti-inflammatory medications, range-of-motion exercises, physical modalities including transcutaneous electrical nerve stimulation as well as superficial ice and heat, and modification and/or restriction of the offending activity. The majority of cases usually have functional resolution within 2 years.

Recovery includes regaining shoulder function and resolution of the scapular winging for most patients, although many are left with a mild degree of endurance limitations in the affected shoulder. When the condition persists despite appropriate conservative management, the patient may be a candidate for surgical management. The surgical procedures for scapular winging generally include scapulothoracic fusion, static stabilization (less favorable), and dynamic muscle transfer (more favorable).

Trapezius palsy due to spinal accessory nerve injury tends to respond less favorably to conservative treatments. Several authors have proposed that if adequate functional recovery has not occurred after 1 year of conservative treatment, then surgery should be considered. Surgical exploration, neurolysis, end-to-end suturing, and nerve grafting have produced variable outcomes but appear to be generally beneficial. The preferred method of treatment for healthy and active patients with isolated chronic trapezius palsy due to spinal accessory nerve injury is the Eden–Lange muscle transfer procedure.

Scapular winging associated with rhomboid paralysis due to dorsal scapular nerve injury is usually mild with minimal functional impairment. Therefore, treatment is usually conservative with cervical spine stabilization (collar or cervical traction), muscle relaxants, anti-inflammatory medications, and physical therapy. Surgical intervention may be indicated in severe cases that fail to respond to conservative treatment.

KEY POINTS TO REMEMBER

- Medial scapular winging, the most common type of scapular winging, results in the medial (spinal) border of the scapula protruding off the dorsal thoracic wall. It is due to weakness of the serratus anterior muscle from damage to the long thoracic nerve.
- Lateral scapular winging is observed as a more lateral displacement of the superior angle of the scapula due to trapezius muscle weakness (injury to the spinal accessory nerve). It can be accentuated by having the individual abduct and externally rotate the arm against resistance.
- Dorsal scapular nerve damage affects the rhomboid muscles, creating a more lateral displacement of the inferior angle.
- Scapular winging may cause significant dysfunction to shoulder mechanics (dyskinesis), affecting certain motions and causing some degree of pain. It is generally managed conservatively.

Further Reading

Berthold JB, Burg TM, Nussbaum RP. Long thoracic nerve injury caused by overhead weight lifting leading to scapular dyskinesis and medial scapular winging. *J Am Osteopathic Assoc.* 2017;117:133–137.

Martin RM, Fish DE. Scapular winging: Anatomical review, diagnosis and treatments. *Curr Rev Musculoskeletal Med.* 2008;1(1):1–11.

Park SB, Ramage JL. Winging of the scapula. *StatPearls.* Treasure Island, FL: StatPearls Publishing. Retrieved September 2019 from https://pubmed.ncbi.nlm.nih.gov/31082049/

Vetter M, Charran O, Yilmaz E, et al. Winged scapula: A comprehensive review of surgical treatment. *Cureus.* 2017;9(12).

7 Burning and Twitching in the Shoulder

Matthew Robinson and Quynh Giao Pham

A 67-year-old female complains of insidious-onset deep ache and burning with weakness of her right shoulder during the past 2 weeks. Rest, ice, and acetaminophen have not helped. She also noticed difficulty lifting her arm and occasional "twitching" over the deltoid. She denies any other neurological symptoms except burning over her thumb. She has a history of a right mastectomy and radiation therapy 6 years ago.

On examination, the mastectomy scar looks intact with mild hyperpigmentation of skin over her right axilla and very mild right arm edema that she reports as chronic and unchanged since soon after her mastectomy. Spurling's test is negative. Passive range of motion of shoulders is normal without focal tenderness and negative impingement maneuvers. Strength is 4/5 in shoulder abduction, elbow flexion, and wrist extensors but otherwise intact. There is reduced sensation to light touch over the deltoid region, lateral forearm, and thumb. Right brachioradialis reflex is absent, but other reflexes are normal.

What do you do now?

The patient complains of mild shoulder pain that is progressive and associated with weakness, without any related injury. The first approach to this case is to determine the etiology of the symptoms. Due to the absence of any trauma and the lack of improvement after resting the limb, local injuries such as rotator cuff tendonitis, bicipital tendonitis, labral tear, osteoarthritis, muscles strain, and bony fractures are less likely etiologies. In addition, examination did not show any pain with local tenderness over the shoulder, and provocative testing for rotator cuff and biceps tendonitis was negative. The presence of burning pain that is not worsened by palpation or range of motion suggests the presence of neuropathic pain.

When considering neuropathic pain, it is important to mentally retrace the nerve pathways from the spinal cord to the peripheral nerves. Neuropathic pain can arise from multiple structures. In the general population, the most common etiologies involve cervical radiculopathy via compression of cervical nerve roots and compression neuropathies of peripheral nerves. Less common etiologies include idiopathic brachial neuritis (IBN), radiation-induced brachial plexopathy (RBP), and compression plexopathy from local mass effect such as neoplastic brachial plexopathy (NBP). Although less common, these etiologies may present with acute-/subacute-onset weakness and shoulder/arm pain. In the case outlined in this chapter, the patient denies any history of neck pain and Spurling's test for cervical compression is negative, making the diagnosis of cervical radiculopathy unlikely. Compression neuropathies often involve dysesthesias along the distal course of the involved nerve. For instance, compression of the median nerve at the carpal tunnel (carpal tunnel syndrome) often presents with symptoms that include dysesthesias of the volar first 3.5 digits and does not involve more proximal distributions of the median nerve. A similar finding is found along the ulnar nerve distribution following compression of the ulnar nerve in the cubital tunnel (cubital tunnel syndrome). These compression neuropathies are less likely diagnoses in this patient because the distribution of neuropathic pain involved both the right deltoid area and portions of the right hand. In addition, Tinel's tests at the carpal and cubital tunnels did not exacerbate the pain, making compression at these sites unlikely. With nerve root compression and peripheral nerve compression lower on the differential, the more appropriate diagnosis would involve the brachial plexus or a diagnosis of brachial plexopathy. Brachial plexopathy from metastatic tumor invasion (NBP) by previous tumor is less likely given the negative positron emission tomography (PET) scan just 1 year prior. However, additional imaging studies of the brachial plexus, such as magnetic resonance imaging (MRI), are warranted and should still be ordered given the patient's history of cancer. IBN or post-radiation plexopathy are more likely but require further diagnostic studies to differentiate between the two. The prognosis is very different, so determining an accurate diagnosis is essential in this scenario (Figure 7.1; Table 7.1).

Idiopathic brachial neuritis, also referred to as Parsonage–Turner syndrome, typically presents with pain and weakness in a brachial plexus-associated distribution. A key characteristic that is identifiable in approximately half of patients who suffer from IBN by a thorough history is a preceding inciting event that typically occurs days to weeks prior to the development of symptoms. This inciting event is typically a physical or emotional stressor such as upper respiratory infection, flu-like syndrome, immunization, surgery, severe anxiety, or a new social stressor. It may also be seen in young athletes engaging in vigorous athletic activities. The etiology of IBN is not entirely understood, and some researchers hypothesize it may be an immune-mediated disorder. As such, it has been reported to manifest bilaterally in up to one-third of patients. Patients will most often present to a provider with abrupt onset of intense neuropathic pain in the affected shoulder/arm/hand. This pain can last anywhere from a few hours to weeks, with spontaneous improvement over time; however, patients will then experience arm weakness. The most commonly affected portions of the brachial plexus are the upper roots and upper trunk. Consequently, weakness may present in the deltoid, biceps, supraspinatus, infraspinatus, and even the serratus anterior,

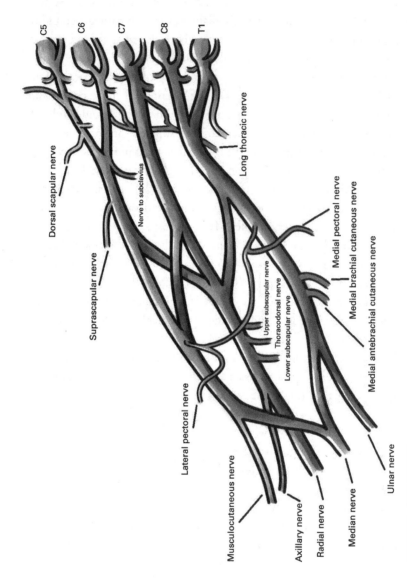

FIGURE 7.1 Brachial plexus.

C5
C6
C7
C8
T1

Dorsal scapular nerve

Suprascapular nerve

Nerve to subclavius

Long thoracic nerve

Upper subscapular nerve

Thoracodorsal nerve

Lower subscapular nerve

Medial pectoral nerve

Medial brachial cutaneous nerve

Medial antebrachial cutaneous nerve

Lateral pectoral nerve

Musculocutaneous nerve

Axillary nerve

Radial nerve

Median nerve

Ulnar nerve

TABLE 7.1 **Differentiating Features of Brachial Plexopathies**

	RBP	IBN	NBP
Brachial plexus trunk affected	Upper	Upper	Lower
Presenting symptom	Dysesthesia + weakness	Severe pain	Severe pain
Best diagnostic modality	EMG	Exclusion	MRI/PET
Causes	Radiation for breast cancer	Physical/emotional stressor	Metastatic breast or lung cancer

EMG, electromyography; IBN, idiopathic brachial neuritis; MRI, magnetic resonance imaging; NBP, neoplastic brachial plexopathy; PET, positron emission tomography; RBP, radiation-induced brachial plexopathy.

leading to some degree of scapular winging. Muscles of the hand and forearm mostly derive innervation from the mid- and lower plexus. Because this is essentially a lower motor neuron process, it is common to observe atrophy of the involved muscles and hyporeflexic or absent deep tendon reflexes of the weakened muscles. Most IBN presentations are incomplete, with a patchy distribution of weakness throughout muscles innervated by the same nerve.

Neoplastic brachial plexopathy is most commonly due to metastasis from a primary breast or lung cancer. Its incidence increases with age. Spread has been reported to be along lymphatics to the axilla and supraclavicular regions in proximity to the brachial plexus. Due to the lymphatic drainage pathways, NBP has a predilection for the lower trunk of the brachial plexus. Consequently, weakness will be reported more distally in the hand/wrist and at times noted in the pectoralis muscles. Like IBN, NBP presents with severe shoulder girdle pain that radiates down to the hand, and mean onset of presentation of symptoms has been reported to be 6 years post surgery. Other etiologies of NBP include a primary lung cancer causing Pancoast syndrome due to its location at the lung apices in proximity to the lower trunk/roots. Classically, Pancoast tumors will show signs of Horner's syndrome (ptosis, miosis, and anhidrosis) in up to 50% of cases.

Radiation-induced brachial plexopathy is a known complication of radiation to the chest, neck, or axillary region. The average onset of symptoms post-radiation has been reported as 6 years, and it is most commonly reported following radiation for breast cancer (40–75% of patients), followed by lung cancer and lymphoma. RBP has also been seen following radiation to treat nasopharyngeal carcinoma with lower cervical lymph node metastases. Studies have found an association between verified cervical lymph node metastasis and development of RBP after radiation.

Unlike IBN and NBP, pain is not consistently reported in this population. Patients may report dysesthesias followed by weakness. In contrast to NBP, RBP has a predilection for upper root/trunk involvement (weakness often involves the deltoid, biceps, supraspinatus/infraspinatus, and serratus anterior). It has been hypothesized that this is in part due to a protective effect of the more superficial clavicle and relatively shorter course of the lower trunk through the radiation beam.

Furthermore, radiation dose, technique, and possibly concomitant chemotherapy may predispose patients to developing RBP. Increased risk of RBP is associated with doses greater than 5600–6000 cGy, larger radiation fields, and two separate courses of subthreshold radiation sessions. Although a clear pathophysiology has not been identified, some postulate radiation leads to microvasculature damage, causing injury to myelin and axons as well as causing extensive perineural fibrosis. Thus, MRI may show thickening and diffuse enlargement of the plexus attributed to this fibrosis. These findings are discussed later but are not specific to RBP. Many features are difficult to distinguish between RBP, IBN, and NBP, but clinical features such as severe pain on presentation and Horner's syndrome can provide clues for early diagnosis.

Typical workup to differentiate the previously mentioned diagnoses includes MRI, PET scans, and electrodiagnostics. MRI is the initial study of choice in the workup of brachial plexopathy, although in cases of trauma, initial plain radiographs may be warranted. MRI has the advantage of being multiplanar, and it has the capability to provide visualization of soft tissue structures. MRI may not help distinguish NBP from RBP because both may show diffuse thickening of the plexus. It will easily differentiate NBP if associated with a tumor mass such as Pancoast tumor impinging the brachial plexus and if the mass is encroaching on the epidural space.

When attempting to differentiate NBP from other plexopathies, PET scan may be warranted following an indeterminate MRI or if MRI is contraindicated. PET scans will localize to areas of high cellular turnover and show intense uptake along the course of involved nerves in the plexus.

Increased uptake is low/minimal in RBP because the pathophysiology is due to a chronic fibrotic process. In contrast, NBP will show significant uptake of the involved plexus and thus is used to identify a metastatic process. In fact, the American College of Radiology has recommended PET as the most appropriate imaging study for use in differentiating RBP from tumor recurrence plexopathy such as NBP.

Electrodiagnostic testing can help differentiate between IBN/NBP and RBP as well as localize the affected nerves. Nerve conduction studies would help confirm the diagnosis of plexopathy and rule out compression neuropathy and peripheral neuropathy. Studies that show relatively intact nerve conduction action potential amplitudes (no significant axonal loss) indicate a better prognosis than those with reduced amplitudes (axonal loss involved). Nerve conduction studies should include more proximal nerves (axillary and musculocutaneous) as well as distal nerves (ulnar, median, radial, lateral, and medial antebrachial cutaneous). Both IBN and RBP have a predilection for the upper trunk, so the ulnar and medial antebrachial cutaneous nerves may be spared. Electromyography (EMG) may show spontaneous abnormal potentials called myokymia, associated with vermicular (worm-like) movement of the skin that may help solidify the diagnosis of indeterminate cases. Myokymia is reported in cases of RBP and not in IBN or brachial plexopathy from tumor invasion. Note that significant fasciculations (muscle twitching that is seen in many chronic neuropathic conditions such as radiculopathy, plexopathy, and compression neuropathy) can be confused with the vermicular motion from myokymia but typically do not have a "writhing" tendency. Myokymia has been noted in 50–70% of patients with RBP, although their presence varies even among muscles innervated by the same portion of the brachial plexus.

Suspecting a neuropathic condition, you request an EMG/nerve conduction study, which reveals significant abnormalities. This patient's clinical picture with a known history of previous radiation treatment and the presence of upper trunk abnormalities on the electrodiagnostic study (including myokymic discharges on EMG) is highly suggestive of post-radiation plexopathy. In the absence of myokymia, the diagnosis of post-radiation plexopathy would have been difficult to differentiate from idiopathic brachial plexus neuritis or plexopathy by tumor compression. The differentiation of these two diagnoses would then be based on the presence or absence of an identifiable mass compressing the plexus on a dedicated brachial plexus MRI.

Radiation-induced brachial plexopathy generally carries a poor prognosis. Most often, patients experience progressive symptomatology leading to profound weakness and disability. It has been reported that approximately two-thirds of patients with RBP experience motor and sensory deficits that worsen over years. The remaining patients show halted progression after up to 3 years. Patients should be advised to continue physical and occupational therapies to maintain functional abilities. There is no clear treatment for this condition, but sometimes lymphatic bypass surgery is attempted to alleviate lymphedema that may be causing a compressive effect on the peripheral nerves.

Idiopathic brachial plexus neuritis generally has a favorable prognosis, with recovery of motor function (sometimes incomplete) over the course of 6–18 months. Recurrence is reported as rare, with no evidence of predisposition to IBN with future physical or emotional stressors. Pain relief can often be achieved with adjuvant analgesics (neuropathic). Pain may be severe enough to prompt immobilization of the limb for short periods of time to prevent flares, but active exercises should be started immediately once the pain starts to improve in order to maintain range of motion of the affected limb. In rare instances, no recovery is seen past 2 years and surgical intervention may be considered. This may include nerve grafting or tendon transfers targeted at functional improvement of shoulder abduction because the upper trunk of the plexus is most often involved.

Neoplastic brachial plexopathy usually carries a poor prognosis and is often managed using palliative measures. Treatments are targeted at decreased tumor bulk with chemotherapy and radiation as well as surgery (tumor debulking). Pancoast tumor interventions involving radiation followed by surgical resection have a 20–35% 5-year survival rate.

KEY POINTS TO REMEMBER

- RBP and IBN usually affect the upper trunk.
- NBP usually affects the lower trunk.
- RBP usually presents with dysesthesias and weakness.

- IBN and NBP usually present with intense pain followed by weakness.
- Symptoms of RBP may not be present for several years (average: 6 years) after the last dose of radiation.
- EMG studies may show myokymic discharges, an abnormal spontaneous activity, which can differentiate RBP from neoplastic and idiopathic plexopathies.
- RBP is most commonly associated with radiation from breast cancer treatment.
- Vermicular movement on the skin (myokymia) can be confused with fasciculations from chronic neuropathic conditions.

Further Reading

Cai Z, Li Y, Hu Z, et al. Radiation-induced brachial plexopathy in patients with nasopharyngeal carcinoma: A retrospective study. *Oncotarget*. 2016;7(14):18887–18895. doi:10.18632/oncotarget.7748

Chandra P, Purandare N, Agrawal A, Shah S, Rangarajan V. Clinical utility of (18)F-FDG PET/CT in brachial plexopathy secondary to metastatic breast cancer. *Indian J Nucl Med*. 2016;31(2):123–127. doi:10.4103/0972-3919.178263

Dropcho EJ. Neurotoxicity of radiation therapy. *Neurol Clin*. 28(1):217–234.

Khadilkar SV, Khade SS. Brachial plexopathy. *Ann Indian Acad Neurol*. 2013;16(1):12–18. doi:10.4103/0972-2327.107675

Kishan AU, Syed S, Fiorito-Torres F, Thakore-James M. Shoulder pain and isolated brachial plexopathy. *BMJ Case Rep*. 2012;2012:bcr0320126100. doi:10.1136/bcr-03-2012-6100

Electricity Running Down the Arm

William J. Molinari, III

A 70-year-old male complains of atraumatic posterior neck pain with electrical shock-like sensations down his arms with neck flexion for 2 months. He additionally reports difficulty performing fine motor tasks such as buttoning his dress shirts or picking up loose change, which he relates to constant numbness and weakness in his hands. He ambulates without an assistive device but admits that walking is more difficult nowadays. His past medical history includes diabetes mellitus.

Focused examination of his arms reveals decreased sensation to light touch through his median, radial, and ulnar nerve distributions and 4/5 motor strength in his deltoid, biceps, and wrist extensors. Biceps reflex is 3+ symmetric (others are normal). Bilateral shoulder active range of motion is slightly limited in all directions but painless. Neck flexion produces a transient experience of focal pain and an uncomfortable "electrical" sensation in both arms. Toe-to-heel walking is challenging.

What do you do now?

Considering the plethora of suggestive nerve-related symptoms on history and physical examination, multiple studies are pursued for further investigation. Cervical spine X-rays demonstrate a loss of normal cervical lordosis with multilevel spondylosis. Non-contrast magnetic resonance imaging (MRI) of the patient's cervical spine reveals significant degenerative disc disease with loss of disc height and disc herniations at C3–C4, C4–C5, and C5–C6, with cerebrospinal fluid signal effacement and significant central canal and neuroforaminal narrowing at the involved levels. Spinal cord signal change, referred to as myelomalacia, is not apparent. X-rays and MRI scans of the patient's shoulders bilaterally are noncontributory.

Cervical radiculopathy (mechanical compression or chemical irritation of one or several cervical spinal nerve roots) often presents with sensory, motor, or mixed deficits in a specific dermatomal pattern correlating to the nerve root(s) involved. These are lesions to the lower motor neuron, not fitting this patient's presentation because dermatomal upper extremity symptoms are not apparent and reflexes were noted to be brisk or normal. These lesions are generally unilateral in contrast to the patient's symptoms, which are bilateral. An MRI of the cervical spine should be ordered to confirm the anatomical pathology as it correlates with history and examination details, along with other tests such as electromyography (EMG) that may help detect physiologic changes affecting cervical myotomes (muscles whose innervation originates from a specific cervical nerve root).

Another consideration in this case could be an idiopathic brachial neuropathy [Parsonage–Turner syndrome (PTS)]. This generally presents as intense unilateral shoulder girdle pain for several days or weeks, followed by motor deficits often without a known precipitating event—hence its name.

Risk factors associated with PTS include a recent viral or bacterial infection, recent immunization, post-surgical state, stress, and trauma to the shoulder girdle (which at times can be relatively trivial). The literature has cited PTS in post-surgical patients from many orthopedic procedures, but also coronary artery bypass, hysteroscopy, and even oral surgery. The incidence of idiopathic brachial neuropathy is 1.6 cases per 100,000 people. However, this is likely underreported due to the difficulty in diagnosing this condition. A formal cervical spine and musculoskeletal workup of the shoulder girdle should be performed to rule out any other contributing or confounding pathology. EMG can also be useful in confirming the suspected diagnosis of PTS because an EMG will show diffuse denervation of muscle groups affected, generally representing several peripheral nerve distributions. Treatment should focus on functional physical therapy combined with nonsteroidal anti-inflammatory drugs for pain. There is little evidence to support the routine use of steroids or alternative treatment modalities such as acupuncture. Opiates should not be considered for initial analgesia.

The constellation of symptoms plaguing the patient in this case are typical of cervical spondylotic myelopathy. The etiology of myelopathy is multifactorial resulting from mechanical cord compression from herniated discs, vertebral osteophytes, dynamic segmental stenosis, and ischemic changes due to compressive forces to the spinal cord vasculature. The incidence of myelopathy in the population increases with age but is likely not truly appreciated due in part to the subtle onset of presenting symptoms, which are often not identified by the patient or physician and are commonly attributed to the normal aging process. In the majority of patients with cervical myelopathy (approximately 75%), their clinical course is often characterized by periods of symptom stability followed by stepwise deterioration. Approximately 20% of patients experience a slow and continual decline in function, whereas 5% experience a rapid onset of symptoms followed by an interval of dormancy.

Cervical myelopathy produces both sensory and motor symptoms, which vary based on the level and location of spinal cord compression. Generalized numbness in the hands can be reported along with subjective weakness and gait instability. Reflexes may be diminished if peripheral neuropathy or cervical nerve root compression is also present. However, cervical myelopathy mainly affects upper motor neurons. Notable upper motor neuron signs are presented in Table 8.1.

Conservative management can and should be tried in cases of cervical radiculopathy, particularly when the evaluation shows soft tissue pathology as the cause of nerve irritation or compression (i.e., herniated disc). Physical therapy modalities, including various types of properly applied cervical traction, superficial heat and cold, and electrical stimulation may help with analgesia and allow the patient to engage in an active exercise program. The patient should be guided through cervical core strengthening exercises and gentle range-of-motion exercises, emphasizing correcting postural imbalances. It is common to see patients with a significant forward head shift. This posture causes undue traction to the cervical roots and the brachial plexus, often leading to dynamic radicular complaints that can be corrected through postural exercises. Cervical epidural steroid injections can be helpful in cases in which a significant inflammatory component is suspected and to achieve some temporary analgesia that may allow the patient to better participate in an active exercise program.

TABLE 8.1 **Upper Motor Neuron Signs in Cervical Myelopathy**

Hyperreflexia	May be diminished if peripheral nerve disease also present.
Hoffmann sign	"Flicking" patient's middle finger distal interphalangeal joint in extension produces flexion of the thumb and index finger.
Inverted brachioradialis reflex	Tapping the brachioradialis tendon along the radial aspect of the wrist elicits finger flexion.
Sustained clonus	Forceful dorsiflexion of the ankle in a relaxed state produces beats of ankle plantar flexion. More than three beats is considered sustained clonus.
Babinski sign/ Plantar Response	Rubbing the lateral aspect of the plantar foot causes great toe extension; may also cause the other toes to flex or curl
Spasticity	Rapid, passive stretch of muscles produces increasing velocity-dependent resistance.

However, in cases in which significant stenosis is detected (centrally or laterally) and in cases in which conservative measures fail to provide relief, surgical intervention should be considered to prevent further neurologic decline and halt the natural progression of myelopathy. The technical aspects of the varying surgical approaches and procedures indicated in myelopathic patients are beyond the scope of this chapter. However, there are many different approaches that depend on the specific pathoanatomical features and the surgeon's expertise/experience. Anterior cervical, posterior cervical, or combined approaches offering both decompression and fusion are commonly performed in these cases. Return to baseline function or reversal of neurologic symptoms should not be expected in cases in which neurological damage has already occurred; the goal is to prevent further neurologic deterioration.

Another important consideration is that in approximately 20% of patients, tandem lumbar stenosis producing lower extremity radiculopathy or neurogenic claudication is also present. This additional pathology is often overlooked or unrecognized as patients and physicians focus on the cervical pathology discovered. If the patient complains of additional lower limb symptoms in the presence of cervical myelopathy confirmed by a cervical spine MRI, then additional evaluation of the lumbar spine may be warranted.

KEY POINTS TO REMEMBER

- Cervical radiculopathy may affect one or more nerve roots in the cervical spine. It often presents as shoulder and arm pain with muscle weakness and sensory symptoms.
- It is important to recognize the symptoms and signs of cervical cord compression versus those of cervical root compression. Cervical cord compression generally features upper motor neuron signs, whereas root compression features lower motor neuron signs. It is also important to realize that both pathologies may coexist, particularly in the setting of chronic spondylosis, causing both central canal stenosis and lateral recess/foraminal stenosis in one or more cervical segments.

- Cervical radiculopathy is a common cause of acute and chronic neck and upper limb pain with neurological deficits.
- MRI of the cervical spine is the imaging modality of choice to assess anatomical pathology, and EMG is the physiological test of choice to detect changes affecting cervical nerve roots and their corresponding myotomes (muscles whose innervation originates from a specific cervical nerve root). Ideally, the clinician should correlate the findings and concordance of these two tests with the patient's history and physical examination findings to reach an accurate diagnosis.

Further Reading

Childress MA, Becker BA. Nonoperative management of cervical radiculopathy. *Am Fam Physician.* 2016;93(9):746–754.

Iyer S, Kim HJ. Cervical radiculopathy. *Curr Rev Musculoskelet Med.* 2016;9:272–280. https://doi.org/10.1007/s12178-016-9349-4

Kjaer P, Kongsted A, Hartvigsen J, et al. National clinical guidelines for non-surgical treatment of patients with recent onset neck pain or cervical radiculopathy. *Eur Spine.* 2017;26:2242–2257. https://doi.org/10.1007/s00586-017-5121-8

Thoomes EJ, van Geest S, van der Windt DA, et al. Value of physical tests in diagnosing cervical radiculopathy: A systematic review. *Spine J.* 2018;18(1):178–189.

9 A Construction Worker Sidelined by Elbow Pain

Bruno Subbarao

A 45-year-old right-handed male construction worker presents with a weeklong complaint of pain in his right elbow. It has been progressively worsening and limiting his ability to perform manual labor. At this point, he has trouble sleeping at night and feels weak in his arm. He found some relief with over-the-counter ibuprofen, but he does not want to take too much because he has had stomach ulcers in the past. He denies any neck pain or numbness or tingling in the arm and hand.

On examination, tenderness is elicited with palpation around the elbow, greatest around the lateral epicondyle. You ask him to extend his wrist against resistance with his elbow in extension, and he reports significant pain at his elbow. Last, you extend his elbow once more and passively flex his wrist down. This time, the patient pulls his arm away in pain, and he massages his elbow for relief.

What do you do now?

- Lateral epicondylitis
- Elbow sprain (lateral collateral ligament) or fracture
- Elbow arthritis
- Cervical radiculopathy
- Olecranon bursitis
- Distal biceps tendonitis
- Radial tunnel syndrome

Epicondylitis is an enthesopathy, a disorder involving the attachment of a tendon or ligament to a bone. It is usually seen in the setting of chronic repetitive microtrauma. Because of repetitive or forceful movements involving motion at the wrist, most commonly extension or supination, a degenerative process caused by the frequent microtrauma will occur within the tendon at its bony attachment. In lateral epicondylitis, also known as "tennis elbow" due to the frequency of this condition seen in recreational tennis players, the extensor carpi radialis brevis (ECRB) muscle is often affected as degeneration encompasses the common wrist extensors origin at the lateral epicondyle (Figure 9.1). In contrast, medial epicondylitis ("golfer's elbow" and "pitcher's elbow") is the analogous condition affecting the attachment of the wrist flexor muscle mass at the medial epicondyle.

At this point, based on the patient's history and physical examination findings (positive findings, lack of a significant trauma history, progression of the complaints, and lack of neurological complaints), we should feel confident that the most likely diagnosis in this case is lateral epicondylitis. Classically, this condition presents much in the same way as described by this patient. Pain is located at the lateral elbow and can often be severe, even causing pain at rest, leading to difficulty sleeping. The pain can cause weakness in grip strength and limit functionality of the limb in its entirety. A progressive, gradual history of increasing pain and weakness is typical.

In suspected cases, physical examination should include inspection and palpation of the painful area but also of the entire arm, as well as the unaffected limb for comparison. Special maneuvers performed on physical

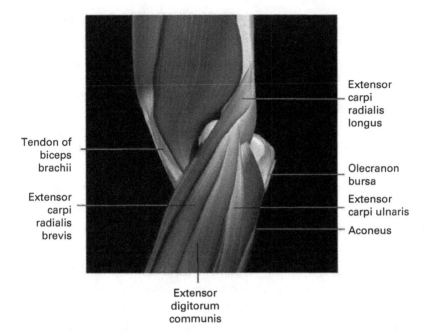

Tendon of
biceps
brachii

Extensor
carpi
radialis
brevis

Extensor
carpi
radialis
longus

Olecranon
bursa

Extensor
carpi ulnaris

Aconeus

Extensor
digitorum
communis

FIGURE 9.1 Anatomy of the lateral elbow.

Reproduced with permission from Hutson, M. A., and Speed, C. *Sports Injuries*. Oxford
University Press, 2011.

examination place stress on the ECRB attachment, eliciting a pain response
that points us toward the diagnosis of lateral epicondylitis (Table 9.1).

Lateral epicondylitis is generally self-limited, with 90% of individuals
recovering within 1 year without treatment. However, this condition could
take up to 18 months for resolution. Thus, initial management should
focus on relative rest, pain control, and assessment and correction of any
improper biomechanics.

The latter recommendation can often be accomplished through referral to an occupational therapist (OT). An OT can also assist with activity modifications, stretching exercises, and education of safe and proper
strengthening techniques. For lateral epicondylitis, eccentric and isometric
strengthening exercises are generally well tolerated, but developing an
individualized home exercise program should be the goal. Finally, OTs can

TABLE 9.1   **Provocative Tests in the Diagnosis of Lateral Epicondylitis**

Test	Description
Cozen's test	Elbow is flexed to 90 degrees, forearm is pronated, and hand is radially deviated. The patient will attempt to extend their wrist under resistance by the examiner. Pain at the lateral elbow is a positive sign.
Mill's test	The provider flexes and pronates the patient's wrist while the elbow is extended. Pain at the lateral elbow is a positive sign.
Maudsley's test	The patient will attempt to extend their middle finger under resistance by the examiner. Pain at the lateral elbow is a positive sign.

provide therapeutic modalities such as icing, electrical stimulation, and myofascial release, and they can recommend bracing options for the patient.

With bracing, there are two common types to consider: a counterforce brace and a wrist extension splint. Counterforce bracing is a forearm strap that, when placed distal to the common wrist extensor mass attachment at the lateral humerus (placed in the proximal forearm), will help transfer biomechanical forces from the common extensor origin to the location of the strap, thus providing relief during activity by dissipating the force at this location. The wrist extension splint is much more restrictive but is meant to keep the wrist in an extended position to allow the extensor tendons to be in a relaxed, shortened state.

Although the braces may be effective in preventing pain, the patient may need some additional pain relief modalities acutely. As mentioned previously, icing is an effective option that can be used multiple times a day for 10–15 minutes at a time. However, if further pain control is needed, options to consider include a topical or oral nonsteroidal anti-inflammatory drug. Topical application may help limit systemic side effects. A third option is an injection of a corticosteroid mixed with an anesthetic into the area of maximal tenderness, which can potentially achieve short-term pain relief for up to a few months.

If initial management is unsuccessful and the patient has completed his course of occupational therapy, it is recommended to re-examine the patient and reconsider the differential diagnosis list for elbow pain. Possibilities include arthritis, fracture, cervical radiculopathy, osteochondritis dissecans, olecranon bursitis, distal biceps tendinitis, lateral collateral ligament sprain, and radial tunnel syndrome.

In general, imaging such as X-rays, magnetic resonance imaging (MRI), or ultrasound evaluation is reserved for cases that do not respond to initial management or if the diagnosis remains unclear. Ultrasound, if available, may be the fastest and most cost-effective means of visualizing the tendon and evaluating for thickening of the tendon, calcifications, osteophytes, tears, and neovascularization (Figure 9.2).

Three-view X-rays of the elbow could help rule out fractures and dislocations while simultaneously demonstrating possible calcifications within the tendon, a sign of chronic repetitive microtrauma. An MRI would be useful in identifying edema and tears and is important in determining if surgery is necessary when symptoms persist beyond 6 months.

If the diagnosis of lateral epicondylitis is confirmed, there should be consideration of nonsurgical treatment options, although many lack a robust

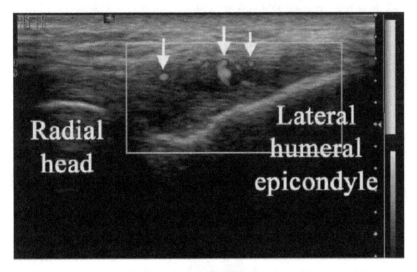

FIGURE 9.2 Ultrasound evaluation to diagnose lateral epicondylitis, demonstrating thickening of the common extensor tendon as well as neovascularization (arrows).

Reproduced with permission from Hutson, M. A., and Speed, C. *Sports Injuries*. Oxford University Press, 2011.

evidence base for support. Therefore, it is important to have an honest conversation with the patient to ensure they are willing and understanding of the risks and benefits. Considering the availability of these procedures and the possibility that insurance carriers may not cover them is important to help the patient with their decision.

A few examples of other nonsurgical treatment options for lateral epicondylitis include tenotomy, platelet-rich plasma (PRP) injections, prolotherapy, and acupuncture. Tenotomy is typically done under ultrasound guidance and is a procedure in which fenestrations are made into the tendon using a needle, followed by injection of an anesthetic and a steroid. PRP injections involve using autologous blood centrifuged to remove red blood cells (and sometimes white blood cells) and then injected in the affected area to supply growth factors released by the activated platelets in an attempt to speed healing of the tissue. Prolotherapy is a procedure in which an irritant, commonly high concentration dextrose, is injected into the affected area, thereby causing inflammation and promoting that the affected tissues utilize their own mechanisms for repair and regeneration. Finally, acupuncture is a popular treatment modality in traditional Chinese medicine, and there is substantial evidence of its effectiveness in the treatment of pain and various musculoskeletal conditions.

For the small percentage of patients who do not respond to any of the previously discussed methods, and whose pain and disability persist beyond 6–12 months, surgery may be warranted. Commonly, surgery will entail debridement of the fibrotic tissue and tendon repair. As with any surgery, there are risks involved, and helping patients formulate appropriate questions prior to their meeting with an orthopedic surgeon is a very helpful way to assist patients in choosing the correct path forward.

KEY POINTS TO REMEMBER

- Lateral epicondylitis is a painful condition caused by chronic repetitive microtrauma and inflammation of the common extensor tendon origin (attachment) located at the lateral epicondyle of the distal humerus.

- Lateral epicondylitis is also known as "tennis elbow" because it is often seen in tennis players due to poor biomechanics and repetitive motions, but it is commonly seen in many other individuals.
- Conservative management after clinical diagnosis is achieved through relative rest, pain control, correction of improper biomechanics, counterforce bracing, and referral to occupational therapy.
- Ultrasound, if available, may be the fastest and most cost-effective means of visualizing the tendon and evaluating for thickening of the tendon, calcifications, osteophytes, tears, and neovascularization.

Further Reading

Brummel J, Baker CL 3rd, Hopkins R, Baker CL Jr. Epicondylitis. *Sports Med Arthrosc Rev.* 2014;22(3):e1–e6. doi:10.1097/JSA.0000000000000024

Sims SE, Miller K, Elfar JC, Hammert WC. Non-surgical treatment of lateral epicondylitis: A systematic review of randomized controlled trials. *Hand.* 2014;9(4):419–446. doi:10.1007/s11552-014-9642-x

Vaquero-Picado A, Barco R, Antuña SA. Lateral epicondylitis of the elbow. *EFORT Open Rev.* 2017;1(11):391–397. doi:10.1302/2058-5241.1.000049

10 A "Golf Ball" in the Elbow

Amir Mahajer, Caitlin M. Cicone, and Melissa Guanche

A 52-year-old right-handed male police officer complains of subacute right elbow pain and swelling during the past 8 weeks. The pain radiates laterally and distally into the forearm, and he reports difficulty with elbow flexion. Elbow flexion and contacting the posterior elbow against objects cause sharp pain. His history and review of systems are otherwise negative. He denies any trauma but reports 4 years of episodic joint pain relieved by rest and over-the-counter medications.

His vital signs are normal. Neurovascular examination is normal. He is guarded and complains of pain with terminal elbow flexion. There is a very large round mass on the posterior right elbow with demarcated erythema. Skin is intact without evidence of a puncture wound or abrasion. The mass is tender to palpation, warm, and fluctuant. There is no elbow instability on stress testing. The remainder of the joints in the upper and lower limbs are unaffected.

What do you do now?

- Tumor, benign (i.e., lipoma) versus malignant
- Septic arthritis
- Elbow fracture
- Bursitis, septic versus aseptic
- Elbow synovial cyst
- Cellulitis
- Inflammatory arthropathy
- Osteochondrosis dissecans versus Panner disease
- Gout and pseudogout
- Epicondylitis, medial or lateral
- Osteoarthritis

Patients with warm, swollen, and erythematous joints are commonly encountered in both the clinic and the emergency room setting. Determining the underlying etiology is imperative because management will differ based on its etiology. Although the case presented in this chapter may suggest an inflammatory arthropathy such as gout, there are other diagnoses that present similarly.

One important concept in this case would be to evaluate for joint red flags. The presence of these would require prompt expeditious action. Red flags include systemic symptoms (fever, chills, fatigue, night sweats, malaise, and/or weight loss) with joint mass/effusion (consider infection or malignancy), significant trauma (consider fracture), joint pain on passive range of motion (consider intra-articular pathology), recent joint/tendon corticosteroid injections (consider tendon rupture or septic arthritis). In immunocompromised individuals or those who meet systemic inflammatory response syndrome (SIRS) criteria, joint or bursa infection must be considered. Evaluation of such patients would require X-rays, blood tests, and aspiration with fluid analysis.

Gout is one of the most common crystal-induced, inflammatory arthropathies. Clinically, it presents when monosodium urate crystals are deposited within a joint or soft tissue, resulting in an inflammatory response. Increased serum uric acid levels (i.e., hyperuricemia) are the primary risk factor for developing gout. Hyperuricemia (serum urate >6.8 or

7.0 mg/dl) may be caused by increased urate production and/or impairment of uric acid excretion. Although all patients who have gout demonstrate high serum uric acid levels, not all individuals with elevated serum uric acid levels will experience a clinically significant event. For those who do experience symptoms from crystal deposition, it has classically been described to occur in three stages: gout flares (acute and episodic arthritis), intercritical gout/recurrent gout flares, and chronic gouty arthritis/tophaceous gout. Acute gout flares are the main focus of this discussion; however, the frequency and duration of gout attacks may increase over time, leading to a chronic condition associated with deposition of uric acid crystals or tophi.

Clinically, acute gout flares present with severe pain, swelling, redness, and warmth of a joint within 12–24 hours. Various dietary and physical factors, comorbid conditions (e.g., hypertension/obesity), and medications (e.g., diuretic use) may provoke a gout flare. In gout flares, often only one joint is involved; however, multijoint involvement may also occur. Although podagra (gout involving the metatarsal–phalangeal joint of the great toe) is the most common site of manifestation, the diagnosis of an acute gout flare should be considered when a sudden, monoarticular arthritis occurs, unless the involved joint is the shoulder. Peripheral joints are most often involved, but involvement of the axial joints can occur (e.g., spine and sacroiliac joints).

The gold standard for diagnosing gout in patients who present with a suspected gout flare involves arthrocentesis and fluid analysis. Fluid analysis should include cell count, differential white blood cell count, gram stain and culture, and examination under polarizing light microscopy. Polarizing light microscopy will demonstrate negatively birefringent crystals in patients with gout flares (sensitivity 85%; specificity 100%). Imaging studies such as X-rays, ultrasound, and magnetic resonance imaging have little utility in the diagnosis of an acute gout flare in the early stages of the disease process, but they may help rule out other causes. Radiographic findings such as subcortical bone cysts or bone erosions due to tophi are more commonly seen in chronic gout and less so in the early disease process (see Figure 10.1 for right elbow radiographs). Ultrasound may identify the mass contents such as rheumatoid nodules or tophi as seen in inflammatory and crystal arthropathies, respectively. Blood tests such as erythrocyte sedimentation rate (ESR), C-reactive protein (CRP), and white blood cell counts are often

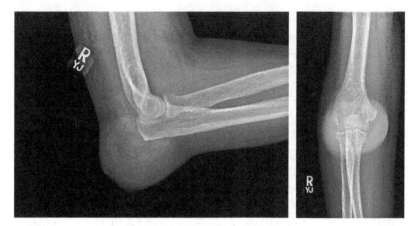

FIGURE 10.1 Right elbow radiographs. A very large tophus with irregular calcifications is observed in the olecranon bursa, without adjacent erosion/destruction of the olecranon process. There is no joint effusion.

Case courtesy of Dr. Matt Skalski (Radiopaedia.org; rID: 29768).

elevated in gout flares. However, many other conditions may also result in elevation of these markers, so they have little diagnostic specificity. The one exception may be in evaluation of a fracture, in which case these values are often normal. In addition, serum uric level during a gout flare can be low or normal, making it difficult to interpret and an unreliable diagnostic tool in the acute setting.

Management of gout is multimodal and involves both pharmacological and nonpharmacological approaches. Both approaches aim to minimize recurrence of gout flares and prevent long-term joint damage.

The natural history of gout flares involves spontaneous resolution, even without treatment. However, with therapy, symptoms improve more quickly, allowing for earlier reduction in pain and disability. The earlier treatment is initiated, the more rapid and completely symptoms resolve. Treatment usually ends 2 or 3 days after symptoms resolve.

After a gout flare, initiation of urate-lowering therapy begins for those with a diagnosis of gout who demonstrate certain features highlighted in Box 10.1. The goal of urate-lowering therapy is to maintain a serum urate level <6 mg/dl. Routine monitoring of serum urate levels is necessary once pharmacological treatment has begun. Typically, urate-lowering treatment begins 2 weeks after a gout flare because starting therapy during a flare may worsen or prolong the inflammatory phase. However, for patients who are already on uric acid-lowering therapy during a flare, treatment should not be discontinued. It is not necessarily recommended that long-term urate-lowering treatment be initiated for all patients after a first gout attack or those with infrequent attacks. For those who are candidates for urate-lower therapy, prophylactic treatment with colchicine or nonsteroidal anti-inflammatory drugs (NSAIDs) may reduce the recurrence of gout flares upon initiation of therapy.

Nonpharmacological management plays an important role in the management of gouty arthropathy and involves identifying reversible causes of hyperuricemia, patient education, and management of comorbid conditions, as shown in Table 10.1. In addition, not all risk factors for gout are modifiable. Nonmodifiable risk factors include age, male gender, menopausal status in females, ethnicity, and genetic variants. Overall, primary goals of nonpharmacological management include patient education, reduction to ideal body weight, dietary changes, dietary supplementation, reducing alcohol consumption, and avoiding/substituting medications that interfere with urate acid metabolism.

An alternative diagnosis is this case is an olecranon bursitis. A bursa is a fluid-filled, sac-like structure lined by synovial membrane. Bursae are located throughout the musculoskeletal system to facilitate movement of other structures. Deep bursae are usually located between bony prominences and muscles or between muscles, and superficial bursae are located between the skin and bone to function as a cushion. Bursitis results from increased fluid production by the synovial cells lining the bursa. Inflammation commonly causes bursitis, increased bursal pressure, and associated pain.

TABLE 10.1 **Nonpharmacological Management**

Patient education	
Identifying reversible causes of hyperuricemia	Dietary factors: unbalanced diets that are high in animal-based purines, sugar-sweetened drinks, low in dietary protein, and alcohol intake
	Medications that impact urate serum levels
Management of comorbid conditions	All of the following are risk factors for gout:
	Hypertension
	Chronic renal failure
	Cardiovascular disease
	Metabolic syndrome
	Obesity
	Hyperlipidemia
	Diabetes mellitus

The most common causes of bursitis include direct trauma, prolonged pressure, overuse, infection (septic bursitis), inflammatory arthritis (rheumatoid arthritis), and crystal-induced arthropathy such as gout.

Acute bursitis presents with tenderness over the bursa and pain with active range of motion of the muscles associated with the bursa as seen in this case; passive range of motion in which the involved muscles are not contracted is normal. Chronic bursitis may present with more swelling in proportion to pain because the bursa has expanded slowly over time and can accommodate the increased intrabursal volumes.

Evaluation of bursitis differs for superficial and deep processes. Forms of evaluation include physical examination, bursal fluid aspiration and analysis, diagnostic imaging, and blood tests.

Physical examination findings for superficial bursitis include swelling, tenderness, and pain with active range of motion. A thorough skin check for puncture wounds or cellulitis is necessary to help rule out infection. Deep bursitis is not usually associated with visible erythema or swelling. Common forms of superficial bursitis include olecranon bursitis (as in this case), prepatellar bursitis, and retrocalcaneal bursitis; forms of deep bursitis include greater trochanteric pain syndrome (formerly trochanteric bursitis), subacromial bursitis, and iliopsoas bursitis.

Bursal fluid aspiration and analysis are indicated to rule out infection and to aide in the diagnosis of a crystal-induced arthropathy such as gout. Fluid analysis should be similar to that done for joint aspirations. Superficial bursitis with erythema and tenderness warrants fluid aspiration to rule out infection, whereas forms of deeper bursitis, such as trochanteric bursitis, rarely do. If septic arthritis or bursitis is suspected, fluid should be analyzed (Table 10.2).

Imaging for superficial bursitis is usually not necessary because physical examination findings usually demonstrate signs of inflammation. For deeper bursitis, imaging may only be necessary when an exact anatomical diagnosis is necessary.

Routine blood work including white blood cell count may be normal in both septic and aseptic bursitis. CRP and ESR are usually elevated in septic bursitis.

TABLE 10.2 **Fluid Analysis**

	Normal	Noninflammatory	Inflammatory	Septic	Hemorrhagic
Clarity	Clear	Clear	Cloudy	Turbid	Bloody
Color	Straw	Straw	Yellow	Yellow/green	Red
Viscosity	High	High	Low	Low	Variable
Mucin clot	Good	Good	Fair	Poor	—
WBCs/mm³	<200	<2,000	2,000–50,000	>50,000	Variable
% PMNs	<25	<25	>50	>75	Variable
Glucose (% serum level)	95–100	95–100	80–100	<50	—
Protein (g/dL)	1.3–1.8	3–3.5	>4.0	>4.0	—
Crystals	None	None	Multiple/none	None	None

PMNs, polymorphonuclear leukocytes; WBCs, white blood cells.

Treatment of bursitis is largely dependent on the underlying etiology and pathology. Septic bursitis is treated with antibiotics, whereas aseptic bursitis is typically treated with anti-inflammatories. Septic bursitis more commonly involves superficial bursa because of the higher predisposition to trauma in these areas. Direct inoculation of bacteria from a puncture wound or spread from adjacent cellulitis is the most common mechanism, hence the importance of a thorough skin check in the evaluation of a superficial bursitis. The most common pathogen associated with septic bursitis is *Staphylococcus aureus*, and it is treated with synthetic penicillins. Along with antibiotics, drainage and surgical debridement may be warranted. Septic bursitis of a deep bursa is less prevalent but can be seen with hematogenous spread or an associated septic joint. The mainstay of treatment in septic bursitis is aspiration, close monitoring, and 10–14 days of oral antibiotics; in immunocompromised patients and those who meet SIRS criteria, hospitalization and intravenous antibiotics are recommended.

Aseptic bursitis management is aimed at alleviating symptoms and preventing secondary complications of immobilization, such as loss of range of motion, muscle atrophy, and joint contracture. An NSAID is the recommended form of analgesia, unless contraindicated. Alternatives for patients with increased risks of NSAID consumption include a selective cyclooxygenase inhibitor or concurrent use of a proton pump inhibitor; for superficial bursitis, a topical NSAID may be considered. An injection of intrabursal local anesthetic and corticosteroid may be considered for deep processes; however, intrabursal steroid injections are not generally recommended for superficial bursitis due to the increased risk for corticosteroid-induced skin atrophy, infection, and local tendon injury. Select patients—athletes and laborers—may benefit from a bursal steroid injection when a rapid return to sport or work is paramount and they have failed to improve with conservative measures.

To prevent secondary complications of immobilization, patients should be educated on the aggravating factors and be given joint protection recommendations. For superficial bursitis such as olecranon bursitis, a firm concave orthosis with a Velcro strap may be useful in shielding the bursa from external pressure. This can be customized by an occupational therapist to ensure range of motion is not limited. Physical therapy for symptomatic relief and stretching/strengthening of the associated musculature in deeper bursitis are recommended. Education on posture and avoiding prolonged pressure over suspected bursa should be part of every treatment plan.

KEY POINTS TO REMEMBER

- Always evaluate and rule out joint and bursa red flags; in the presence of red flags, act expeditiously.
- For suspected fractures, elbow X-rays (anteroposterior, lateral, and radial head views) should be obtained and the joint immobilized in a posterior long arm splint, 45–90 degrees of elbow flexion with neutral wrist.
- In suspected septic arthritis/bursitis, obtain appropriate blood studies, aspiration, and fluid analysis; consider consultation with orthopedic surgeon and infectious diseases specialist.
- The gold standard for diagnosis of a crystal-induced arthropathy, such as gout, involves arthrocentesis and fluid analysis. Under polarizing light microscopy, negatively birefringent crystals are visualized.

Further Reading

Baumbach SF, Lobo CM, Badyine I, Mutschler W, Kanz KG. Prepatellar and olecranon bursitis: Literature review and development of a treatment algorithm. *Arch Ortho Trauma Surg*. 2014;134(3):359–370.

Chand A, Pobre T. Olecranon bursitis. In: Kahn SB, Xu RY, eds. *Musculoskeletal Sports and Spine Disorders: A Comprehensive Guide*. Cham, Switzerland: Springer; 2017:97–100.

Qaseem A, Harris RP, Forciea MA; Clinical Guidelines Committee of the American College of Physicians. Management of acute and recurrent gout: A clinical practice guideline from the American College of Physicians. *Ann Intern Med*. 2017;166:58.

11 The Case of the Burning Pinky

Quynh Giao Pham

A 60-year-old female complains of worsening pain in the fourth and fifth digits of her left hand of gradual onset during the past 4 months. She also describes tingling and burning sensation worse toward the end of the day. She is a hair stylist, and her left hand fatigues easily with prolonged gripping of the hair dryer.

Neck, shoulder, wrist, and finger examinations reveal normal painless range of motion. There is tenderness of the left ulnar groove and medial epicondyle. Tinel's test over the left elbow elicits pain in the forearm as well as the fourth and fifth fingers. Resisted wrist flexion and passive wrist extension caused pain over the medial epicondyle but no pain in the fourth and fifth digits. Tinel's test over the wrist is negative. Focused neurological examination is normal except for slight atrophy of the left first dorsal interosseous. Sensation was reduced over dorsal and palmar aspects of the left fourth and fifth digits.

What do you do now?

- Is there a neurological injury?
- Could there be an elbow overuse injury?

This patient presents with pain that is likely neuropathic (tingling and burning sensation) in the fourth and fifth digits. The innervation to this area is the ulnar nerve, supplied by the lower trunk of the brachial plexus and derived from the C8/T1 nerve roots. Thus, the lesion is likely somewhere along this nerve pathway (Figure 11.1), and the differential diagnosis for the symptoms from distal to proximal includes ulnar nerve compression at Guyon's canal, the cubital tunnel, and the ulnar groove; brachial plexus compression at the upper trunk (thoracic outlet syndrome); and nerve root compression at C8/T1 (radiculopathy). Before reviewing the possible cause of this patient's neuropathic symptoms, we should ensure that local causes of the burning pain are ruled out, including local skin irritation or infection such as cellulitis.

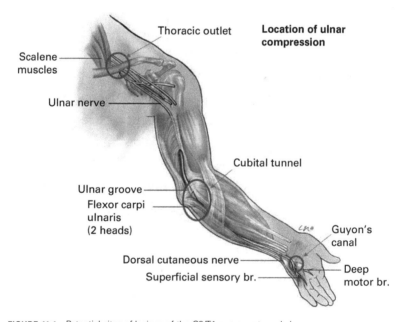

FIGURE 11.1 Potential sites of lesions of the C8/T1 nerve roots and ulnar nerve.

Ulnar nerve compression at Guyon's canal usually presents with pain-less weakness of the intrinsic hand muscles. The roof of Guyon's canal is formed by a ligament between the hook of the hamate and the pisiform. As the ulnar nerve crosses under this canal, a branch of the dorsal cutaneous nerve exits above the canal and thus can be spared if the main ulnar nerve is compressed within the canal. Therefore, patients with this compression may notice intrinsic hand weakness, but usually without sensory changes. Ulnar nerve compression at Guyon's canal occurs when constant pressure is applied over the ulnar aspect of the wrist (e.g., constant tight grip of a bicycle's handlebar) or when there is direct trauma (e.g., martial arts chop). In this patient, there is no noted trauma to the wrist, and the presence of sensory symptoms and signs makes this diagnosis less likely.

The most common site of ulnar nerve compression is over the retrocondylar (ulnar) groove of the distal humerus and the cubital tunnel (between the two heads of the flexor carpi ulnaris). The ulnar groove is the area between the medial epicondyle and olecranon where the ulnar nerve travels as it crosses the elbow. The ulnar groove is covered by a retinaculum (ligament arcuatum or Osborn ligament), which also contributes to the compression of the ulnar nerve. The nerve continues to travel distally through the fascia of the cubital tunnel, between the two heads of the flexor carpi ulnaris. These two locations are next to each other, and most references to cubital tunnel syndrome refer to ulnar nerve compression at the cubital tunnel and/or ulnar groove.

Ulnar nerve compression at the cubital tunnel/ulnar groove presents with pain or paresthesias and numbness over the fifth and fourth digits and weakness of the ulnar-innervated intrinsic muscles (interossei, lumbricals, and hypothenars). In addition, tapping over the ulnar nerve at the ulnar groove (Tinel's test) may not only cause tenderness but also reproduce the sensory symptoms in the fingers. Although symptoms of ulnar nerve com-pression in these two areas are very similar, the pathology is quite different. Compression of the ulnar nerve across the ulnar groove occurs with re-petitive pressure over this area (resting on a hard surface) or excessive and prolonged elbow flexion, which results in stretching of the ulnar nerve. Treatment of this includes elbow cushion and sleeve to prevent further nerve compression and avoidance of excessive elbow flexion. On the other hand, ulnar nerve compression over the cubital tunnel can occur with edema, injury, hypertrophy, or pressure over the flexor carpi ulnaris. The treatment for this includes icing, stretching of the flexor muscle, and allowing the nerve to rest and heal.

Other sites of ulnar nerve injury include compression at the lower trunk of the brachial plexus. These injuries can occur from trauma (e.g., overstretching of the brachial plexus when hanging from a bar with one arm), Klumpke's palsy, or local compression from a cervical rib or tight scalene muscles (thoracic outlet syndrome). Symptoms are similar to those of cubital tunnel syndrome but with additional sensory abnormality in the medial forearm due to involvement of the medial brachial cutaneous nerve and also additional weakness involving all intrinsic hand muscles, including thenar muscles (supplied by the median nerve). Because the brachial artery travels together with the lower trunk, testing for compression of the artery (Adson's test) can help establish the diagnosis of nerve compression at this location. The test is performed with the examiner palpating for the radial pulse with the patient's arm at rest and then again with the arm in abduction, externally rotated, and slight extension (elbow extended). The patient is then asked to turn the head toward the ipsilateral side. The test is positive for neurovascular compression if the pulse is diminished or absent. Depending on the cause of the injury, treatment may include surgical resection of the scalene, removal of cervical ribs, etc.

Last, irritation of the C8 and T1 nerve roots (radiculopathy) will also present as neuropathic pain in the fourth and fifth fingers. The most common cause of nerve root impingement is neuroforaminal stenosis at the C7/T1 level due to disk herniation or facet arthropathy. Other causes include spondylolisthesis and mechanical compression from a cyst, hematoma, and tumor. Unlike plexus lesions, nerve root lesions will affect the paraspinal muscles, which are innervated by the posterior ramus, a branch off the nerve root soon after it exits each neural foramen. Patients with C8/T1 radiculopathy will often have cervical spine pathology and compression of the neuroforamina with neck extension, and rotation toward the affected side (Spurling's test) may reproduce pain in the fourth and fifth fingers. The symptomatic management of cervical radiculopathy is multimodal and includes medication management for neuropathic pain, including antiepileptic medication, antidepressants, as well as anti-inflammatory medication such as nonsteroidal anti-inflammatory drugs (NSAIDs), or a short course of corticosteroids. Physical therapy can be instituted with cervical stabilization exercises, posture training, and cervical traction if the spine is stable. Interventional procedures such as epidural steroid injections can also help alleviate the pain temporarily. If muscle weakness is progressive, surgical decompression may be indicated.

The patient in this case presents with burning pain, tingling sensation in the fourth and fifth fingers (palmar and dorsal aspect), accompanied by some atrophy of the first dorsal interosseous. In addition, the pain is reproducible with Tinel's test over the ulnar groove. These findings suggest that the lesion is over the ulnar nerve as it courses through the ulnar groove, or cubital tunnel syndrome. Due to the presence of sensory abnormality in the dorsal fourth and fifth digits, a lesion at Guyon's canal is less likely because sensory supply to this area via the dorsal cutaneous nerve would have been spared. Ulnar lesion proximal to the elbow is also less likely because the patient does not have any pain complaint or sensory abnormality over the medial forearm. In addition, both Adson's test (for thoracic outlet syndrome) and Spurling's test (for cervical radiculopathy) are negative (Table 11.1).

Nerve conduction and electromyography can be done to confirm the diagnosis of nerve entrapment. Findings of slowed conduction velocity of the ulnar nerve in the segment across the elbow compared with forearm segment would confirm entrapment in the cubital tunnel or ulnar groove. Ulnar motor conduction to the first dorsal interosseous muscle may be a more sensitive test in borderline cases. In addition, nerve conduction study can detect the presence of axonal loss, suggesting a more advanced lesion and a poorer prognosis. Given that the patient has atrophy of the first dorsal interosseous muscle, axonal loss is an expected finding, heralding a poorer prognosis. Additional testing to include electromyography of ulnar-innervated muscles (first dorsal interosseous and hypothenar muscles) can help in determining severity of the lesion and prognosis. Findings of active denervation in the muscle suggest ongoing (active) nerve damage, and findings of reinnervation suggest chronicity of the condition. Testing of muscles that are supplied by other nerves (e.g., the median nerve) in the C8/T1 myotomes can help determine if concomitant pathology in the cervical nerve roots, such as radiculopathy, is present.

The diagnosis of cubital tunnel syndrome is primarily made by history and physical examination, confirmed by electrodiagnostic study. Mechanical

TABLE 11.1 **Conditions That May Present as Ulnar Nerve Entrapment**

Location	Condition	Nerve Affected	Sensory Changes	Motor Changes	Pertinent Examination
Above elbow	Brachial plexopathy	Median nerve (from C8/T1 roots) Medial antebrachial cutaneous branch Ulnar nerve	Medial forearm Medial half of fourth digit and fifth digit (dorsal and palmar)	Weak FCU, hypothenar, interossei, lumbricals forearm pronation Benediction sign, thenar weakness	Pain over medial supracondylar area
Elbow	Cubital tunnel compression	Ulnar nerve—all branches including dorsal ulnar cutaneous branch	Medial half of fourth digit and fifth digit (dorsal and palmar)	Benediction sign Weak FCR, FDP Pronator quadratus thenar weakness	+Tinel's test over pronator teres muscle
Wrist	Guyon's canal compression	Ulnar nerve—deep motor branch and superficial sensory branch (sparing dorsal ulnar cutaneous branch)	Medial half of fourth digit and fifth digit (palmar only)	Thenar muscles except adductor pollicis brevis	+Tinel's test over the wrist

FDP, flexor digitorum profundus; FCR, flexor carpi radialis; FCU, flexor carpi ulnaris.

compression is usually the cause. If symptoms are mild, the condition is often self-limiting and no further workup will be needed. Rarely, if tumor, scarring, cyst, or bony deformity are suspected in the nerve compression, imaging such as plain films or magnetic resonance imaging may be helpful. Ultrasound has also been used to assess the degree of nerve compression, but its usefulness as a single diagnostic tool has not been fully established.

In the majority of cases, cubital tunnel syndrome carries a good prognosis, and most patients improve with conservative management. If the condition is mild, with intermittent symptoms and nerve conduction showing only sensory nerve involvement without any axonal loss, treatment consists of elbow bracing/padding to alleviate pressure over the elbow and to prevent excessive flexion of the elbow, which can cause traction on the nerve. NSAIDs can help reduce swelling, and medications such as gabapentin can help alleviate the neuropathic symptoms. Ultrasound-guided corticosteroid injections to the elbow have not been shown to offer additional symptomatic improvement compared to placebo. The condition is considered severe if the symptoms progressively worsen, with hand weakness and muscle atrophy. In such cases, patients should be counseled in seeking more aggressive interventions such as surgical decompression of the nerve. Delay in treatment can result in permanent nerve damage and significant loss of hand function. Prior to any aggressive surgical interventions, it is important to ensure that diagnoses such as cervical radiculopathy, brachial plexopathy, and peripheral neuropathy are ruled out because these conditions can present with similar symptoms.

KEY POINTS TO REMEMBER

- Cubital tunnel syndrome is the most common compression neuropathy affecting the ulnar nerve.
- Cubital tunnel syndrome commonly presents with sensation abnormalities in the fourth and fifth digits, with positive Tinel's sign at the elbow.
- Cubital tunnel syndrome can arise from ulnar nerve compression at the ulnar groove or between two heads of the flexor carpi ulnaris muscle proximally.

- Cervical radiculopathy at the C8/T1 level and lower trunk brachial plexopathy may present with similar symptoms.
- The presence of muscle atrophy and complaints of hand weakness should prompt more aggressive treatment.

Further Reading

Assmus H, Antoniadis G, Bischoff C, et al. Cubital tunnel syndrome—A review and management guidelines. *Cent Eur Neurosurg.* 2011;72(2):90–98.

Caliandro P, La Torre G, Padua R, Giannini F, Padua L. Treatment for ulnar neuropathy at the elbow. *Cochrane Database Syst Rev.* 2016;11(11):CD006839.

Chen IJ, Chang KV, Wu WT, Özçakar L. Ultrasound parameters other than the direct measurement of ulnar nerve size for diagnosing cubital tunnel syndrome: A systemic review and meta-analysis. *Arch Phys Med Rehabil.* 2019;100(6):1114–1130.

Landau ME, Campbell WW. Clinical features and electrodiagnosis of ulnar neuropathies. *Phys Med Rehabil Clin North Am.* 2013;24(1):49–66.

Lleva JMC, Chang KV. Ulnar neuropathy. *StatPearls.* Treasure Island, FL: StatPearls Publishing; 2019. Retrieved June 4, 2019, from https://www.statpearls.com/articlelibrary/viewarticle/30739.

VanVeen KE, Alblas KC, Alons IM, et al. Corticosteroid injection in patients with ulnar neuropathy at the elbow: A randomized, double-blind, placebo-controlled trial. *Muscle Nerve.* 2015;52(3):380–385.

12 A Very Strong Woman with an Achy Forearm and Weak Grip

Quynh Giao Pham

A 49-year-old female complains of right forearm pain and hand weakness for 2 months. She first noticed a deep aching pain in the forearm during an intense workout. Pain subsequently resolved, but it returned intermittently and is now nearly constant. She describes it as a deep ache in the volar forearm and associated with tingling of the first three digits. She claims that her grip is now weaker, and she has cramps when playing tennis.

Examination reveals tenderness over her anterior forearm, and pain is reproduced with resisted forearm pronation. Sensation is reduced in the first three digits and thenar eminence. Grip strength is weaker on the right. She has difficulty making the "OK" sign with the thumb and index fingers. Wrist flexion shows slight ulnar deviation, but wrist extension is normal. Reflexes are symmetric and preserved bilaterally. Tinel's tests at the wrist and elbow, shoulder impingement tests, Spurling's test, and Adson's test are negative.

What do you do now?

- Is there a neurological injury?
- Could there be a muscle overuse injury?

This patient presents with local pain in the forearm and sensory and motor deficits on examination. The presence of local tenderness in the forearm helps localize the pain area. In addition, pain is worse with resisted pronation, suggesting that the muscle tendon or muscle causing this movement may be involved. The muscle mass in the anterior forearm, just distal to the elbow, consists of the wrist flexors, of which only the pronator teres contributes to pronation. The patient also complains of weakness in her grip, and on examination, the distal joint flexion of the first three digits is weak, possibly suggesting a lesion to either the respective tendons or the respective muscle(s) nerve supply. In this case, a nerve injury is more likely due to the sensory abnormalities and weakness (nerve injury that involves both motor and sensory components).

Review of the upper limb anatomy shows that the innervation of the anterior/medial forearm is supplied by the ulnar and the median nerves. The ulnar nerve supplies motor innervation to the flexor carpi ulnaris, long finger flexors for the fourth and fifth digits [flexor digitorum profundus (FDP)], and most intrinsic hand muscles except most of the muscles comprising the thenar eminence. Because the patient's weakness involves the first three digits, sparing the fourth and fifth digits, ulnar nerve pathology as well as C8/T1 pathology are unlikely to contribute to the current symptoms. The median nerve innervates the flexor carpi radialis (FCR), the flexor digitorum superficialis (FDS), long finger flexors to the second and third digits (FDP), most thenar muscles, and the first and second interossei. Thus, it is most likely that the median and/or a branch of the median nerve is involved. Because the weakness extends to muscles that are proximal to the wrist, proximal median entrapment is most likely the cause of this patient's symptoms.

The median nerve has contributions from ventral roots of C5 to T1 and receives contributions from the lateral and medial cords of the brachial plexus. It courses through the arm between the biceps and brachialis muscles to the elbow, where it gives off an articular branch and a branch to the pronator teres muscle before entering the elbow joint. In some individuals, a band of thick connective tissue that stretches from the humeral supracondylar process to the medial epicondyle (ligament of Struthers) is present, and the median nerve crosses under this structure on its way to the elbow. After giving off the branch to the pronator teres, it passes through the bicipital aponeurosis (lacertus fibrosus) and travels between two heads of the pronator teres, giving off branches to supply the FCR, palmaris longus, and FDS. While still within the pronator teres, it gives off a larger branch, the anterior interosseous nerve (AIN), before continuing its course to the wrist. The AIN is a pure motor branch providing innervation to the pronator quadratus, the flexor pollicis longus (FPL), and the radial half of the FDP that controls distal phalanx flexion of the index and middle finger (Figure 12.1). Proximal compression of the median nerve and its branches can occur at the pronator teres and, less commonly, at the ligament of Struthers, lacertus fibrosus, and the fibrous arch of the origin of the FDS muscle. Lesions directly affecting the AIN result in a motor neuropathy (weakness of the FDP, FPL, and pronator quadratus) with no sensory deficits. This condition is referred to as anterior interosseous syndrome (also known as Kiloh–Nevin syndrome) and can occur from radial or supracondylar fractures, tight fibrous bands, and tight or injured pronator teres. Patients typically present weak pronation and inability to flex the distal phalanges of the index finger and thumb to make the "OK" sign. The patient described here has sensory symptoms in the hand and forearm; thus, anterior interosseous syndrome is unlikely to be the diagnosis.

The presence of pain over the pronator teres helps localize the area of involvement. Injury or repeated pressure over the pronator teres can compress the median nerve as it passes through it before giving off the branch of the AIN. If this occurs, the median nerve and all its branches distal to the pronator teres will be affected. Similar to the anterior interosseous syndrome, the etiology of the impingement is generally due to injury of the pronator teres from repetitive muscle strain, overuse or hypertrophy, or hematoma or tumor in this area. It most commonly occurs in women aged 40–50 years, especially those who perform forceful or repetitive forearm pronation. Pronator teres syndrome often presents with pain in the anterior forearm; sensory deficits (numbness, tingling, and burning) in the entire

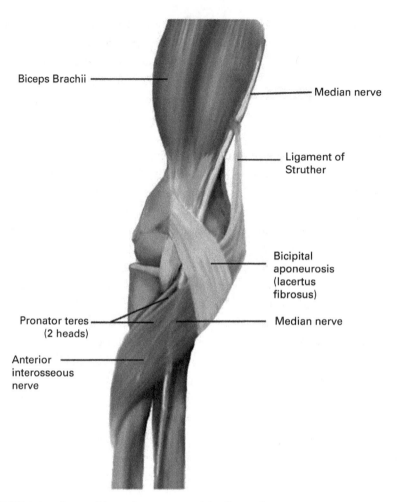

Biceps Brachii

Median nerve

Ligament of
Struther

Bicipital
aponeurosis
(lacertus
fibrosus)

Pronator teres
(2 heads)

Median nerve

Anterior
interosseous
nerve

FIGURE 12.1   Course of the median nerve around the elbow region.

cutaneous distribution of the median nerve in the hand; and some degree of weakness of the FPL, pronator quadratus, thenar eminence muscles, FDS, and FDP. Patients with this condition will have difficulty making a fist due to inability to flex the first three digits (referred to as the Benediction sign). Median nerve compression at the lacertus fibrosus presents similarly to pronator teres syndrome because the two locations are very close. The main difference is that symptoms of median compression by lacertus fibrosus will be worse with resisted elbow flexion and/or supination (contracting the biceps) because the lacertus fibrosus arises from the biceps, whereas symptoms of median compression by the pronator teres will be worse with resisted pronation (contracting the pronator teres).

Pronator teres syndrome shares some of the features of carpal tunnel syndrome (CTS) and can mimic this condition. One crucial difference is that the sensory deficits in pronator teres syndrome involve the thenar area of the palm, an area that is typically spared in CTS. The other clues are weakness involving proximal muscles such as FPL and FDP and, to a lesser degree, pain extending proximally to the forearm, although proximal pain is relatively common in CTS. Because the pronator muscle attaches at the medial epicondyle, this syndrome can be associated with medial epicondylitis. Further testing for this condition involves tapping or applying pressure (Tinel's test) over the pronator teres or contracting the muscle with resisted pronation and observing for reproduction of symptoms. In some patients, pronator teres syndrome occurs concurrently with CTS, making the diagnosis more challenging. Because the treatment for each condition is different, it is important to make the correct diagnosis.

Electrodiagnostic studies are very helpful for confirming the diagnosis of peripheral nerve compression and differentiating between pronator teres syndrome, AIN syndrome, and CTS. In anterior interosseous syndrome, routine sensory and motor testing of the median nerve will be normal, whereas denervation on electromyography (EMG) may be noted only in three muscles (the FPL, part of the FDP, and the pronator quadratus), sparing the thenar muscles. In pronator teres syndrome, median nerve sensory and motor testing will be abnormal, and EMG testing generally shows sparing of the pronator teres muscle but denervation of all distal median innervated muscles. In CTS, muscles proximal to the wrist will not be affected. Imaging studies such as magnetic resonance imaging and ultrasound can further assist in localization of the area of compression and evaluation of the morphology of the nerve.

Treatment of pronator teres syndrome includes conservative measures such as stretching and gentle massages of the pronator teres muscle. Control of swelling in the muscle with activity limitation, frequent ice application, arm elevation, and nonsteroidal anti-inflammatory drugs can be helpful as well. Overall, the prognosis for proximal median entrapment neuropathy

TABLE 12.1 **Median Nerve Injuries and Findings by Anatomical Location**

Location	Condition	Nerve Affected	Sensory Changes	Motor Changes	Pertinent Examination
Above elbow	Ligament of Struthers compression	Median nerve including Anterior interosseous nerve Palmar cutaneous branch	First 3½ digits and thenar area	Weak forearm pronation Benediction sign Weak FCR, FDS, FDP, thenar muscles	Pain over medial supracondylar area
Elbow	Pronator teres syndrome	Median nerve including Anterior interosseous, Palmar cutaneous branch	First 3½ digits and thenar area	Benediction sign Weak FCR, FDS, FDP, pronator quadratus, thenar muscles	+Tinel's over pronator teres muscle
	Anterior interosseous syndrome	Anterior interosseous nerve	None	Weak FPL, FDP, pronator quadratus	Hand weakness without pain
Wrist	Carpal tunnel syndrome	Median nerve, sparing palmar cutaneous branch	First 3½ digits	Thenar muscles except adductor pollicis brevis	+Tinel's over the wrist

FCR, flexor carpi radialis; FDS, flexor digitorum superficialis; FDP, flexor digitorum profundus; FPL, flexor pollicis longus.

without weakness or findings of axonopathy on EMG/nerve conduction study is good, and most patients do well with conservative treatment. Anterior interosseous syndrome carries a good prognosis as well, and most cases resolve spontaneously. However, if the condition persists more than 6 months or progresses involving muscle weakness, more aggressive interventions such as local injection with corticosteroids or surgical decompression may be indicated. The prognosis after surgical decompression is satisfactory, with some recovery of weakness.

The patient discussed in this chapter presents with pain in the anterior forearm that is worse with active resisted pronation. This hints to the possible location of the injury. The pain is accompanied by complaints of burning pain and sensory deficits over the median innervated area on examination, suggesting a neuropathic origin. Examination findings of weakness of distal finger flexors of the first to third digits are similar to those found in CTS, but negative Tinel's test over the wrist and sensory changes over the thenar area of the palm are consistent with a median nerve lesion proximal to the wrist. The presence of sensory symptoms essentially rules out anterior interosseous syndrome as a cause. Ligament of Struthers compression is also not likely due to absence of pain with pressure over the medial epicondyle. Because this patient has pain with resisted pronation and not with elbow flexion, pronator teres syndrome (rather than lacertus fibrosis) is the likely diagnosis (Table 12.1).

KEY POINTS TO REMEMBER

- Proximal median nerve compression can occur concurrently with CTS.
- Anterior interosseous syndrome presents with pure motor deficits, and patients will have difficulty making the "OK" sign.
- Pronator teres syndrome presents with both pain and weakness in the forearm and sensory abnormalities in the first 3½ digits and thenar area.
- Although rare, median nerve compressions at the ligament of Struthers and bicipital aponeurosis (lacertus fibrosus) can occur and may be confused with medial epicondylitis.

Further Reading

Caetano EB, Sabongi Neto JJ, Vieira LA, Caetano MF, De Bona JE, Simonatto TM. Struthers' ligament and supracondylar humeral process: An anatomical study and clinical implications. *Acta Ortop Bras.* 2017;25(4):137–142.

Dididze M, Sherman AI. Pronator teres syndrome. *StatPearls.* Treasure Island, FL: StatPearls Publishing; 2019. Retrieved January 28, 2019, from https://www.statpearls.com/articlelibrary/viewarticle/27808.

El-Haj M, Ding W, Sharma K, Novak C, Mackinnon SE, Patterson JMM. Median nerve compression in the forearm: A clinical diagnosis. *Hand.* 2019 [Epub ahead of print].

Lee, M, LaStayo P. Pronator syndrome and other nerve compressions that mimic carpal tunnel syndrome. *J Orthop Sports Phys Ther.* 2004;34(10):601–609.

Rodner CM, Tinsley BA, O'Malley MP. Pronator syndrome and anterior interosseous nerve syndrome. *J Am Acad Orthop Surg.* 2013;21(5):268–275.

Wertsch JJ, Melvin J. Median nerve anatomy and entrapment syndromes: A review. *Arch Phys Med Rehabil.* 1982;63(12):623–627.

13 Can't Sleep While Hands Are Taking a Nap

Ramon Cuevas-Trisan

A 47-year-old female complains of gradually worsening pain in the wrists for approximately 3 months. She denies any trauma and does not recall any precipitating event. She is known to have a history of hypothyroidism of about 3 years of evolution. She is a homemaker and is slightly overweight, having gained approximately 8 pounds during the past year.

Upon further questioning, she confirms that there are occasional hand paresthesias and some numbness, worse at night, occasionally waking her up. When asked about what part of the hand has the numbness and paresthesias, she states "the whole hand."

She has taken acetaminophen and over-the-counter ibuprofen intermittently when the pain gets more severe. This generally helps relieve some of the pain but does not help the other symptoms.

The hands have a symmetric normal appearance. Grip strength appears to be normal bilaterally and so does gross sensation to light touch. There is no tenderness to palpation.

What do you do now?

- Is this a neurological problem or a soft tissue/musculoskeletal problems with some vague neurological symptoms?
- Could this be a focal manifestation of a systemic condition?
- What additional history details should you seek and what additional workup should you perform?

The time course of this patient's presentation along with the lack of trauma and an essentially normal examination suggest that there is no major anatomic disruption. The possibility of an overuse syndrome that has gradually worsened is the most likely scenario. There are many possibilities, from a chronic condition such as wrist osteoarthritis to soft tissue pathology (ligament/tendon sprain/strain) or a focal neurological problem such as an entrapment neuropathy. Her sensory complaints along with a preexisting underlying condition (hypothyroidism) raise suspicion of a focal neuropathy of the median nerve [carpal tunnel syndrome (CTS)]. However, the reported normal examination casts some doubt about this diagnosis. Another important diagnostic consideration is a cervical radiculopathy. This diagnosis can even be more important to consider when there is more proximal symptomatology (i.e., pain along the arm extending proximally into the elbow, shoulder, periscapular region, or neck), something not uncommonly seen in patients with CTS. A cervical radiculopathy may present abnormalities in reflex testing in the arm, which would not be expected in CTS. Osteoarthritis and CTS often present bilaterally, whereas cervical radiculopathies tend to be unilateral.

Additional examination maneuvers could help narrow the differential diagnosis. Simple tests such as Tinel's test (percussion with a reflex hammer over the distal wrist at the level of the transverse carpal ligament in the midline), Phalen's test (passively holding the wrist in full flexion for 45–60 seconds), and carpal compression tests (compression by examiner over the carpal tunnel for 30 seconds) should be performed. Tinel's test would be considered positive if it results in radiating pain/paresthesias distally into the palm and/or fingers. It has been reported to have a sensitivity between 40% and 90% and specificity of 55–100%. An unusual but important variant would be the patient reporting retrograde or proximal radiation of symptoms upon Tinel testing. This is called the valleix phenomenon, and it is rare yet highly specific for a diagnosis of CTS. Phalen's test would be considered positive if it reproduces the symptoms reported by the patient. Its sensitivity and specificity have been reported to be between 40% and 85% and 54–98%, respectively.

Grip strength and cursory sensory testing is not uncommonly reported as normal, particularly in cases of early/mild CTS. Manually testing the strength of the abductor pollicis brevis can provide information about functional impairment, but it is difficult to assess in most cases on the basis of clinical examination alone when the weakness is not profound. Pin sensation on sensory examination tends to be quite subjective, but monofilament testing adds some degree of objectivity and can be used to map out sensory loss. Abnormal 2-point discrimination (along with vibratory sensation loss) is a later manifestation usually seen in cases of more severe nerve injury. One important factor to consider when evaluating sensation is the cutaneous sensory distribution of the median nerve. As the median nerve crosses the carpal tunnel, the nerve divides into a motor portion (recurrent motor thenar branch and motor branch to the first two lumbricals) and the digital sensory branches, supplying the palmar aspects of the thumb, index, middle, and radial half of the ring finger. The skin over the thenar eminence receives cutaneous innervation from the palmar cutaneous sensory branch of the median nerve, typically given off by the main trunk of the median nerve just proximal to entering the carpal tunnel (Figures 13.1 and 13.2). Therefore, sensation over the palm (over the thenar eminence) is usually spared in CTS. One sign that may be apparent with advanced median nerve injury is the observation of thenar atrophy (indentation or hollowing of the thenar mound). This is usually a late sign accompanying weakness and implies severe CTS. Some clinicians believe that it may be too late to operate once the nerve damage has reached this state.

Imaging studies are usually not necessary because they will generally yield no useful information. Exceptions to this are evolving techniques such as magnetic resonance imaging (MRI) tractography and ultrasonography. Diagnostic ultrasonography can show an enlarged cross-sectional area of the nerve proximal to the entrapment location. The most reliable ultrasonographic measurement is to obtain the cross-sectional area of the median

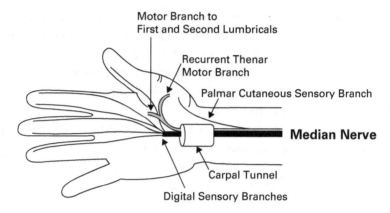

FIGURE 13.1   Distal branches of the median nerve.

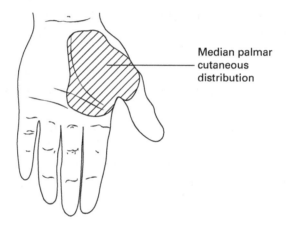

FIGURE 13.2   Cutaneous distribution of the median palmar cutaneous nerve.

nerve on transverse imaging at the wrist and distal forearm typically measured at the level of the pisiform. MRI may also be useful if a structural or
space-occupying lesion is suspected, but there is no specific correlation with
the median neuropathy, and the expense usually outweighs the value of this
type of testing.

The best test to consider in this situation is electrodiagnostic testing.
The test should be performed by an experienced and well-trained specialist
(generally a physical medicine and rehabilitation specialist or a neurolo-
gist) and will generally consist of the nerve conduction portion, including

surface electrical stimulation of the median nerve along its path in the palm through the forearm and elbow, as well as perhaps other nerves (radial and ulnar) for comparison purposes. Most often, there will be no need to do an electromyogram (use of a needle electrode inserted into some of the muscles of the hand and forearm), although this may be necessary in the more advanced/severe cases as detected by the nerve conduction study in order to assess whether the nerve damage has caused damage to the nerve axons, indicating a more advanced and severe lesion.

This patient has a few risk factors for CTS, including her gender, her history of hypothyroidism, being overweight, and her age. The first step in the management of most CTS cases is conservative. This includes the use of nighttime wrist splints that hold the wrist in neutral to slight extension. If the symptoms are more pronounced and also occur frequently during the day, using the splints during the daytime may be recommended. Dorsal splints are also available to facilitate use of the hands during the daytime. The use of diuretics and nonsteroidal anti-inflammatory drugs can also be considered. Splints should be consistently used for no less than 6–8 weeks. Medications should be used for at least 3 or 4 weeks. Simultaneously, the patient should be instructed to get some relative rest of the hands—that is, be aware of avoiding excessive use of the hands, as much as possible.

For more advanced cases or those in which the more conservative measures are not effective, corticosteroid injections into the carpal tunnel could be considered. These injections work by delivering a potent anti-inflammatory agent around the median nerve, at the site of entrapment, thus reducing some of the chronic inflammation that further contributes to increased pressure on the nerve and some of the symptoms. This is a relatively simple office-based procedure that requires no special patient preparation such as fasting or sedation. It is now commonly performed using ultrasound guidance to visualize the nerve and vessels in order to avoid accidentally damaging these. However, in experienced hands, the procedure may be performed without visualization using only anatomical landmarks. An alternative intermediate approach could be the use of phonophoresis (therapeutic ultrasound modality typically administered by a physical or occupational therapist) with dexamethasone. When combined with splint use, it has been shown to provide better results than splinting alone. There are also some studies showing the effectiveness of therapeutic laser treatment compared to placebo.

Ultimately, if the previously discussed measures are ineffective or in cases of more severe nerve entrapment, surgery should be considered. Surgery consists of simply cutting the transverse carpal ligament. This ligament is the "roof" of the carpal tunnel on the volar side of the wrist. By cutting it, more room is created for all the contents of the tunnel, most notably the median nerve, decreasing the pressure over it. Two general surgical approaches can be used: arthroscopic and open releases. The arthroscopic release technique has the obvious advantage of being less traumatic, creating a much smaller set of incisions, and faster postoperative recovery compared to the open approach, in which a longer skin incision is made over the volar aspect of the wrist, fully visualizing and exposing the ligament, followed by transection; this can also be done via a minimally invasive approach using a shorter wrist incision. Of note, a higher rate of accidental median nerve damage has been reported in some of the arthroscopic series, presumably due to poorer intraoperative visualization field. A potential severe complication is the development of complex regional pain syndrome, reported in up to 5% of cases in some series.

Conservative and surgical approaches have both shown improved clinical outcomes, but surgical decompression seems to provide better long-term effectiveness. However, nonsurgical management should be tried initially unless there are severe or persistent symptoms.

KEY POINTS TO REMEMBER

- CTS is the most common entrapment neuropathy in adults; it affects women more than men, and symptoms are generally reported to gradually worsen after insidious onset.
- Common conditions that cause systemic neuropathies (diabetes and hypothyroidism) or edema (pregnancy and renal insufficiency) are risk factors for the condition. In addition, obesity has been described as a risk factor for this condition. Repetitive wrist motion (e.g., in secretarial work) and use of

vibrating tools (e.g., in some construction jobs) are considered occupational risk factors for the condition.
· Patients with mild CTS will usually present symptoms with either no signs or relatively minor signs on examination.
· Electrodiagnostic testing is the only ancillary test that will be useful in confirming the diagnosis. It will also provide the degree of nerve compromise, helping guide possible interventions.
· Conservative followed by more invasive management methods may be used for management in a stepwise manner.

Further Reading

D'Arcy CA, McGee S. The rational clinical examination. Does this patient have carpal tunnel syndrome? [published correction appears in *JAMA*. 2000;284(11):1384]. *JAMA*. 2000;283(23):3110–3117.

MacDermid JC, Wessel J. Clinical diagnosis of carpal tunnel syndrome: A systematic review. *J Hand Ther*. 2004;17(2):309–319.

Padua L, Coraci D, Erra C, et al. Carpal tunnel syndrome: Clinical features, diagnosis, and management. *Lancet Neurol*. 2016;15:1273–1284.

Sucher BM, Schreiber AL. Carpal tunnel syndrome diagnosis. *Phys Med Rehabil Clin North Am*. 2014;25:229–247.

Wipperman J, Goerl K. Carpal tunnel syndrome: Diagnosis and management. *Am Fam Phys*. 2016;94(12):993–999.

14 Wrist Pain After Slip and Fall

Amanda Spielman,
Anne-Sophie Lessard, and
Sriram Sankaranarayanan

A 20-year-old right-hand-dominant female comes to the emergency department after slipping on a wet floor and falling on an outstretched hand (FOOSH injury). She presents with pain and swelling over her right wrist. She describes worsening pain when rotating or bending her wrist sideways. She denies any numbness or paresthesias but believes that her grip is weak.

On physical examination, there is no gross deformity, but there is evidence of some inflammation. There is ulnar-sided wrist pain (tenderness to touch) and some weakness noted as diminished grip strength. There are no sensory deficits or alterations noted. Also noted is stiffness with decreased wrist range of motion attributed to pain.

What do you do now?

- Is there a wrist fracture?
- Could there be a wrist sprain instead? If so, is there a triangular fibrocartilage complex (TFCC) tear, a lunotriquetral (LT) ligament injury, or a scapholunate ligament (SLL) injury?
- Is this a case of a wrist contusion?

In the evaluation of traumatic injuries, imaging studies are paramount. The wrist is a very complex structure, and its radiographic evaluation requires very specific views. The following is a summary of the basic plain radiographs that should be obtained with this presentation.

X-rays are ordered and do not show any evidence of fractures (Figure 14.1). Suspecting the possibility of a soft tissue injury, the patient is placed on a splint, referred to a hand specialist, and conventional magnetic resonance imaging (MRI) is then ordered to evaluate the presence of soft tissue injury.

DISCUSSION

Based on the patient's presentation and initial negative plain radiographs, the most likely diagnosis is a TFCC sprain. Wrist fractures, particularly those affecting the carpal bones, may be difficult to detect initially using plain films and can commonly present as "occult" fractures.

An SLL injury generally presents with dorsoradial-sided wrist pain. This is a different site of tenderness than the one presented in this patient. However, SLL injuries should be considered because 5% of all wrist sprains involve the SLL. Patients with these injuries often report a "click" or snapping of the wrist, swelling, limited grip strength, and reduced range of motion.

The SLL allows for smooth rotation of the wrist by providing stability to the proximal carpals, ensuring the scaphoid and lunate bones move together. Injury may cause abnormal wrist alignment depending on the severity of the disruption.

Clinical examination includes use of Watson's test to determine the presence of a complete SLL injury. This scaphoid stability maneuver is

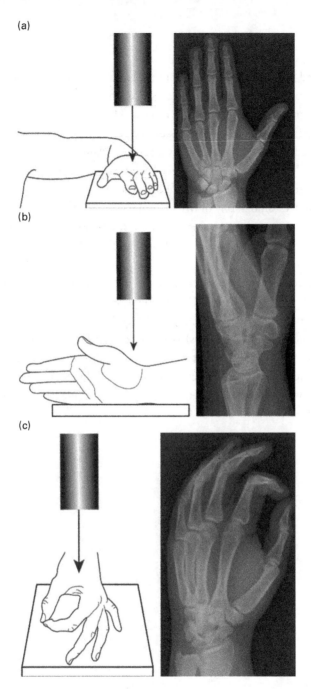

FIGURE 14.1 Standard views of anteroposterior, lateral, and oblique are imaged. (a) Frontal view: arm is flexed 90 degrees and affected hand is placed palm down on the image receptor. All joints in transverse plane, perpendicular to central beam. (b) Lateral view: arm flexed at 90 degrees. Patient abducts humerus to position parallel to receptor. All joints aligned in transverse plane, perpendicular to central beam. (c) Oblique view: affected hand is placed palm down on the image receptor. Shoulder, elbow and wrist are placed in transverse plane, perpendicular to central beam. Wrist is externally rotated 40–45 degrees from PA projection.

performed by grasping the wrist from the radial side and placing the thumb on the scaphoid prominence on the palmar side of the patient's hand while simultaneously holding the distal fingers. The examiner moves the wrist radially with constant thumb pressure (Figure 14.2). The examination is determined positive with instability and pain. Plain films may show a possible Terry Thomas sign on anteroposterior view, which is a gap between the scaphoid and the lunate of more than 3 mm.

Computed tomography or MRI may assist in diagnosis, but arthroscopic exploration is necessary to stage injury and address prognosis. Diagnosis may be challenging due to delayed presentation of instability between 3 and 12 months.

Untreated SLL injuries may progress to arthritic complications and abnormal joint mechanics. Often, unless accompanied by a fracture, conservative treatment involving wrist splints and nonsteroidal anti-inflammatory drugs (NSAIDs) is sufficient. Arthroscopic repair should be performed on total SLL tears within 4–6 weeks following trauma. Surgical treatment involves debridement of torn ligament fibers to allow for regrowth and reattachment in severe cases followed by casting or splinting.

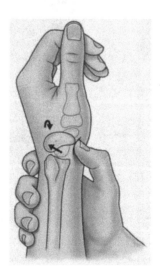

FIGURE 14.2 Watson's test.

Another possible diagnosis is an LT ligament injury. The LT ligament is an interosseous carpal ligament providing intrinsic stability to the proximal carpal row. The LT ligament is composed of a dorsal, intermediate, and strong volar region. The volar component is the major contributor to the functional stability of the LT ligament. An intact LT ligament is required for wrist mobility and range of motion.

Lunotriquetral ligament injuries are an uncommon cause of ulnar-sided wrist pain and similarly caused by a FOOSH. These injuries may also occur when the hand is forced into pronation when lifting. Isolated LT injuries are rare and therefore represent a diagnostic challenge due to comorbid conditions. The proximity of structures in the region often delays a precise diagnosis. Often, extrinsic ligaments are also involved, such as the ulnotriquetral ligament and dorsal and volar radiolunotriquetral ligaments.

Patients typically report ulnar-sided wrist pain, worsening with rotation, reduced grip strength, and tenderness over the LT joint. Several tests can be used to examine the wrist. One of the most useful ones, the Reagan test, is performed by stabilizing the lunate and the examiner identifies pain or crepitus while translating the triquetrum. The Kleinman test is used to identify the presence of laxity (Figure 14.3). In this test, the examiner applies dorsal force to the pisiform and triquetrum and volar force to the lunate.

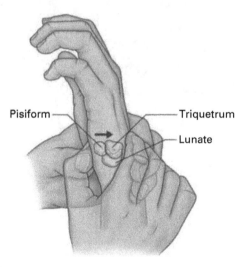

FIGURE 14.3 Kleinman test.

Posteroanterior radiographs are also taken to examine the LT space and, occasionally, MRI studies are used to provide information on the state of intrinsic ligaments. Arthroscopy is the gold standard diagnostic imaging for LT ligament injuries.

Lunotriquetral ligament injuries are first treated with immobilization to ensure proper alignment during healing. NSAIDs can also be used. Unstable injuries can be treated with arthroscopy, and depending on the severity, surgical repair may be required to establish proper alignment and repair damage to the ligament.

As indicated previously, the most likely injury in this case is a TFCC sprain. The TFCC is the fibrocartilage and ligamentous tissue that supports the distal radioulnar joint, originating from the distal radius and ulnar heads and stretching to the proximal carpal bones (Figure 14.4). The complex consists of the ulnotriquetral ligament, meniscal homologue, articular disc, dorsal radio ulnar ligament, volar radio ulnar ligament, ulnolunate ligament, and the ulnar collateral ligament.

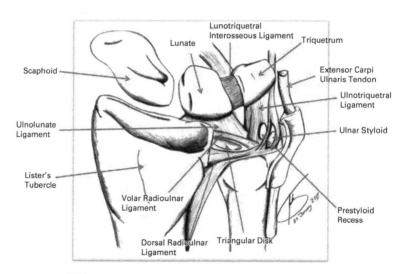

FIGURE 14.4 TFCC anatomy.

Source: Chong (2013).

Injury to this complex is most often caused by a specific injury such as FOOSH with forearm pronation. TFCC sprains can also result from chronic injury such as repetitive heavy loads on the wrist often seen in athletes. Class 2 TFCC injuries have a degenerative etiology, with prevalence of injury increasing with age.

Key findings on physical examination include ulnar-sided wrist pain when gripping and tenderness at the prestyloid recess. There may also be a fovea sign (tenderness on the fovea region, which is a soft spot bounded dorsally by the ulnar styloid, proximally by the ulnar head, volarly by the flexor carpi ulnaris, and distally by the pisiform) and pain over the ulnar aspect of the wrist on wrist ulnar deviation (TFCC compression) or radial deviation (TFCC tension).

Plain films do not contribute to the detection of TFCC sprains or tears and are usually negative, unless there are fractures to surrounding bones (hook of hamate, ulnar styloid, base of fifth metacarpal, and triquetrum distal radius). Fractures will present with swelling or deformity and are generally seen in cases of significant trauma.

MRI can detect a tear at the ulnar part of lunate, but arthroscopy is the gold standard for diagnosis and indicated following nonresponsiveness to splinting after several months.

Treatment involves immobilization with wrist splinting depending on the severity of the sprain and use of NSAIDs for pain. Patients should be advised to follow the RICE protocol: rest, ice (apply 15 to 20 minutes at a time), compression (utilize a bandage to manage swelling), and elevation. Athletes should follow the protocol for 4 weeks. If there is no detectable joint instability, rest with immobilization should be followed with re-examination after 1 week. Corticosteroid injections may also help. Arthroscopy is used to classify TFCC injury, and surgical treatment with debridement and repair is useful for more severe injury or tears. Surgical treatment is determined based on the staging of the injury as noted in Table 14.1.

TABLE 14.1 **Palmar Classification of TFCC Injuries**

Class 1

Traumatic injury	Treatment
1A: Central perforation	1A: Debridement
1B: Ulnar TFCC disruption with or without distal ulnar fracture	1B: Surgical repair; partial tears treated arthroscopically
1C: Distal TFCC disruption	1C: Arthroscopy and debridement
1D: Radial TFCC disruption with or without sigmoid notch fracture	1D: Arthroscopy and debridement Surgical reattachment, partial resection via arthroscopy

Class 2

Degenerative injury, as determined by degree of intact LT ligament	Treatment
2A: TFCC wear	2A–2C: Conservative treatment
2B: TFCC wear with lunate or ulnar chondromalacia	
2C: TFCC perforation, lunate or ulnar chondromalacia	
2D: TFCC perforation, lunate or ulnar chondromalacia, LT ligament perforation	2D: Shaft-shortening with osteotomy
2E: TFCC perforation, lunate or ulnar chondromalacia, LT ligament perforation, ulnocarpal osteoarthritis	2E: Resection of ulnar head

LT, lunotriquetral; TFCC, triangular fibrocartilage complex.

KEY POINTS TO REMEMBER

· Wrist sprains comprise 25% of athletic injuries and are diagnosed based on location and knowledge of detailed anatomy, as well as the degree of instability. TFCC tears are reported as the most common ligament injury, followed by SL then LT tears. SL and LT ligament injuries are often seen in injured TFCC wrists and should be considered when TFCC tears are diagnosed.

- Radial-sided wrist pain lends to a diagnosis of SLL injury often caused by hyperextension and supination of the wrist. Pain is localized to the space between the third and fourth extensor compartments, and disruption can cause dorsal intercalated segment instability. Imaging may show the presence of widening between the scaphoid and lunate in the presence of an SLL tear.
- Ulnar-sided wrist pain may be caused by TFCC sprains or tears and less commonly LT ligament injuries. TFCC injuries also present with tenderness to palpation, a possible "click" with rotation of the forearm and distal radioulnar join instability. LT ligament injury presents with volar intercalated segment instability.
- Treatment and patient adherence to treatment recommendations are necessary to prevent chronic wrist pain, instability, and degenerative arthritic conditions. Conservative treatment options are used involving ice, wrist splints or wraps, and NSAIDs. Gold standard diagnosis is conducted through arthroscopic exploration to determine severity, prognosis, and required surgical intervention. Recovery rates are considered excellent with proper and timely treatment.

Further Reading

Andersson JK. Treatment of scapholunate ligament injury: Current concepts. *EFORT Open Rev.* 2017;2(9):382–393. doi:10.1302/2058-5241.2.170016

Avery DM, Rodner CM, Edgar CM. Sports-related wrist and hand injuries: A review. *J Orthop Surg Res.* 2016;11(1):99.

Geissler WB, Burkett JL. Ligamentous sports injuries of the hand and wrist. *Sports Med Arthrosc Rev.* 2014;22(1):39–44.

Ricolescu R. Ouellette E, Kam C. The incidence of scapholunate, lunotriquetral and triangular fibrocartilage complex tears: A cadaveric investigation. *Orthopedic Proc.* 2018;96-B(11).

15 Skateboarder Hand Blues

Sriram Sankaranarayanan and Amanda Spielman

A 25-year-old male comes to the emergency department after a fall from his skateboard with pain and swelling over his right wrist. He describes landing on concrete, breaking the fall with his right hand. He was not wearing a helmet or other protective gear but denies any trauma to the head, neck, or shoulder. He clearly recalls the entire incident.

The patient is otherwise healthy with no contributory past medical history. His arm is somewhat achy, but he denies any numbness or paresthesias.

On physical examination, both hands have superficial abrasions. There are no neurovascular deficits or deformities other than significant swelling and tenderness to palpation over the right hand's anatomic snuffbox. Range of motion of the wrist is markedly limited due to pain, and axial loading of the hand is very painful. Plain films of the right wrist were obtained. These did not show any obvious fractures.

What do you do now?

· Is there an occult wrist fracture?

· Is this a case of a wrist contusion?

· Could there be a wrist sprain instead?

Occult carpal fractures are common and, in this case, based on the significant trauma and examination findings should be highly suspected. The frequency of these fractures is depicted in Figure 15.1.

Scaphoid fracture is one of the most common upper limb injuries. It is the most common carpal bone to be fractured, constituting 60–70%

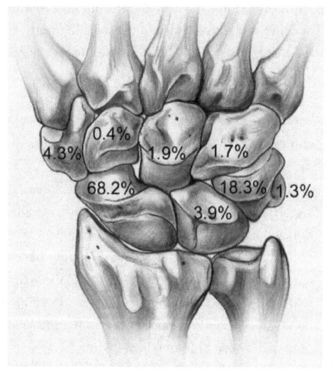

FIGURE 15.1   Frequency of carpal bone fractures.

of all carpal bone fractures. It accounts for up to 15% of acute wrist injuries.

These fractures are more common in younger individuals as a result of a fall on an outstretched hand (FOOSH injury). In older individuals with a FOOSH injury, the distal radius is more commonly fractured.

The presentation commonly involves pain over the anatomic snuffbox (Figure 15.2) and tenderness volarly over the area of the scaphoid tubercle (Figure 15.3).

Initial plain films in the setting of a scaphoid fracture may be unremarkable, with reported false-negative rates of up to 20%. If these are negative but there is a high index of clinical suspicion, a computed tomography (CT) scan or magnetic resonance imaging (MRI) scan may be obtained. These have high specificity and sensitivity in diagnosing occult scaphoid fractures.

The mainstay of treatment is immobilization with a short thumb spica cast. Any suspicion of scaphoid fracture without radiologic evidence should be casted. Scaphoid fractures usually require prolonged immobilization.

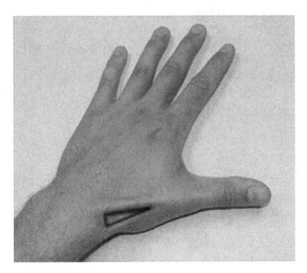

FIGURE 15.2   Pain over anatomic snuffbox.

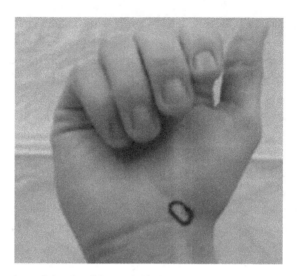

FIGURE 15.3 Anatomic location of the scaphoid tubercle.

The recommended duration of immobilization depends on the location of the fracture along the scaphoid bone (Figure 15.4) as follows:

Distal pole: 4–6 weeks
Waist: 10–12 weeks
Proximal: 12–20 weeks

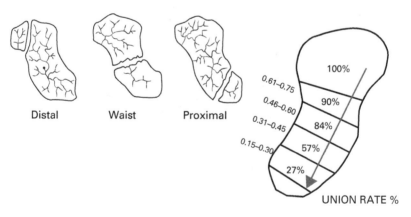

FIGURE 15.4 Scaphoid anatomy and union rates based on location.

The scaphoid receives a tenuous blood supply, and the patient must be educated about the possibility of non-union or avascular necrosis, especially in more proximal fractures.

One feared complication of these fractures is a scaphoid non-union advanced collapse manifested by advanced collapse and progressive arthritis of the wrist. Referral to a hand specialist is important, especially in the following situations:

- Displaced fracture more than 1 mm
- Fractures with scapholunate ligament injury
- Delayed presentation including evidence of non-union or osteonecrosis
- Proximal pole fractures of scaphoid (higher risk of non-union and osteonecrosis)
- High-demand patients with a desire to return to work or sports earlier
- Any pain at the snuffbox area with negative X-rays

Regarding surgical management, most proximal pole fractures require surgery. Distal pole surgery depends on the type of fracture. Surgery can be performed using open or percutaneous approaches.

The second most common carpal bone to be fractured is the triquetrum, accounting for up to 15% of all carpal fractures. Patients present with a history of FOOSH injury and pain along the dorsal ulnar aspect of the wrist. These fractures are most often identified in the oblique or lateral radiographs. As with other carpal fractures, a CT scan may be indicated if initial plain films are inconclusive. The most common fracture pattern is a dorsal cortical fracture (chipped bone displaced dorsally). Most triquetrum fractures are treated initially with a volar splint with the wrist in slight extension leaving the metacarpophalangeal joints free. Once the swelling subsides (generally 1 or 2 weeks), a cast may be applied for a total of 4–6 weeks of immobilization. Referral to a hand specialist is important for assessment and follow-up, but surgery is rarely needed; it is mainly considered for displaced body fractures.

Another relatively common fracture is that of the hook of the hamate (Figure 15.5). These have an incidence of only 2% of all carpal bone fractures but are common in individuals who play sports such as golf,

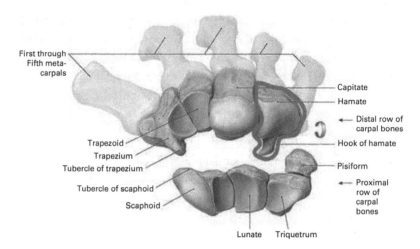

First through
Fifth meta-
carpals

Trapezoid
Trapezium
Tubercle of trapezium
Tubercle of scaphoid
Scaphoid

Capitate
Hamate
Distal row of
carpal bones
Hook of hamate
Pisiform
Proximal
row of
carpal
bones

Lunate   Triquetrum

FIGURE 15.5 Hook of hamate and body of hamate.

tennis, and baseball/softball, in which the end of a golf club, racquet, or bat is forced into the palm, exerting direct pressure on the hypothenar area. Patients often present with a sports injury with pain along the volar ulnar aspect of the wrist. Pain on gripping is frequently reported. The ulnar nerve is in close proximity to the hook of the hamate, and the presentation may include signs of ulnar nerve compression such as decreased sensation in the ring and little fingers and/or impaired motor function of the intrinsic hand muscles along with decreased grip strength. On examination, there is also tenderness along the hook of hamate. This can be assessed as follows: The pisiform bone is a prominent bone located on the ulnar aspect just distal to the wrist crease. After palpating the pisiform, the examiner should place the thumb 1 or 2 cm distal at a 45-degree angle. The hook of hamate is appreciated as a small bony prominence between the index and middle fingers.

The carpal tunnel view in plain films is most useful in detecting hook of the hamate fractures. In this view, the wrist is dorsiflexed approximately 135 degrees, making the carpals and metacarpals lift away from the cassette. Conservative management generally involves a volar resting splint for several weeks. Early referral to a hand specialist is recommended because the management of these injuries is still controversial, ranging from 6 weeks of immobilization to excision of the fractured fragment or screw fixation.

. Scaphoid fractures (and other carpal bone fractures) are often missed on initial X-rays. With a high degree of suspicion, a CT scan or MRI scan can be useful to diagnose an occult scaphoid fracture. Thumb spica splint is the initial management modality. The scaphoid has tenuous blood supply, and often prolonged immobilization may be necessary for fracture healing. Early referral to a hand specialist is recommended.

. Triquetrum fractures often present with pain and tenderness on the ulnar and dorsal aspect of the wrist. They are usually treated nonoperatively with immobilization for 4–6 weeks.

. Hook of hamate fractures are common in golfers and baseball players. They present with pain over the hook of hamate area and sometimes with ulnar nerve dysfunction symptoms. Immobilization with a volar splint is the initial line of management, followed by 6 weeks of immobilization. Surgical intervention includes excision of the fractured fragment or screw fixation.

Further Reading:

Alshryda S, Shah A, Odak S, et al. Acute fractures of the scaphoid bone: Systematic review and meta-analysis. *Surgeon*. 2012;10:218.

Bachoura A, Wroblewski A, Jacoby SM, et al. Hook of hamate fractures in competitive baseball players. *Hand*. 2013;8:302.

Balci A, Basara I, Çekdemir EY, et al. Wrist fractures: Sensitivity of radiography, prevalence, and patterns in MDCT. *Emerg Radiol*. 2015;22:251.

Carpenter CR, Pines JM, Schuur JD, et al. Adult scaphoid fracture. *Acad Emerg Med*. 2014;21:102.

Eastley N, Singh H, Dias JJ, Taub N. Union rates after proximal scaphoid fractures: Meta-analyses and review of available evidence. *J Hand Surg Eur*. 2013;38:888.

Urch EY, Lee SK. Carpal fractures other than scaphoid. *Clin Sports Med*. 2015;34:51.

Wong K, von Schroeder HP. Delays and poor management of scaphoid fractures: Factors contributing to nonunion. *J Hand Surg Am*. 2011;36:1471.

16 Thumb Pain That Keeps Getting Worse

Julio A. Martinez-Silvestrini

A 75-year-old right-handed male with a known history of left hip osteoarthritis (status post total hip replacement) complains of right thumb pain for the past year. He denies trauma. He points to the base of his right thumb as the area of pain and discomfort. He describes intermittent localized swelling in the area. He denies any numbness or tingling.

On physical examination, the patient has localized tenderness and swelling in the area of the first right carpometacarpal joint. There is no redness or increased temperature to palpation. He has full active range of motion and can open and close his hand without sensation of locking of his fingers or thumb. There is normal strength on the right hand. Axial compression of the first carpometacarpal joint causes pain. Ulnar deviation of the wrist does not cause thumb pain. If he clenches his fist with his thumb inside his fist, he has pain on the area of the first carpometacarpal joint. There is no tenderness to palpation on the lateral (radial) aspect of his wrist. The rest of the neuromuscular physical examination appears normal.

What do you do now?

- Carpal tunnel syndrome
- "Gamekeeper's" thumb
- "Trigger" thumb
- De Quervain's tenosynovitis
- Carpometacarpal osteoarthritis

Carpal tunnel syndrome (CTS) is one of the most common ailments affecting the wrist and hand. The patient denies any numbness or tingling, making the possibility of CTS less likely. Patients with CTS usually report numbness on the first three digits (thumb, index finger, and middle finger). Some patients may complain of numbness on the ulnar or lateral aspect of the fourth digit (ring finger). It is common for patients with CTS to complain of numbness or tingling at night, while driving, or while holding a phone. Approximately 50% of patients with CTS have bilateral symptoms. In patients with hand numbness, electrodiagnostic studies, also known as nerve conduction studies and electromyography, should be considered.

"Gamekeeper's" thumb is an injury to the ulnar collateral ligament of the thumb. It usually occurs traumatically with forced abduction of the thumb. Radiographs are recommended in cases of significant trauma. In the absence of trauma, the possibility of an acute ligament injury is much less likely.

This patient's physical examination failed to show any locking or catching of his thumb, excluding the possibility of a "trigger" thumb. In this condition, a localized swelling or nodule is formed on the flexor pollicis longus tendon causing a characteristic locking of the thumb at the interphalangeal joint. This is typically painful while trying to extend the thumb from a flexed position. Although the locking sensation appears to occur at the interphalangeal joint, the pathology occurs at the thenar eminence.

De Quervain's tenosynovitis is a subacute to chronic tendon inflammation or tendinosis of the first dorsal wrist compartment, comprising the abductor pollicis longus and extensor pollicis brevis tendons. It is usually the result of overuse or cumulative injuries of the wrist with the thumb extended. It occurs most commonly in women aged 30–50 years. Finkelstein's test is the diagnostic maneuver used to make this diagnosis. Interestingly, since 1958, several textbooks have confused this maneuver with a similar test, Eichhoff's test. Finkelstein's test is performed by the patient actively deviating the wrist ulnarly and then the examiner passively flexing the thumb (Figure 16.1b). Eichhoff's test is performed by the patient clenching their thumb, followed by passive ulnar deviation of the patient's wrist by the examiner (Figure 16.1c). Eichhoff's test appears to cause more discomfort and have a lower specificity (89% vs. 100%), but in the author's clinical experience it is still a very useful maneuver.

Most of the medical evidence suggests that in the treatment of de Quervain's tenosynovitis, the combination of injected corticosteroids and bracing using a thumb spica (cast or brace) is superior to injection or bracing alone. There is no significant difference when comparing conservative care in the form of hand therapy and injection, but in patients who are significantly disabled by their pain, injections followed by hand therapy are recommended. A multi-modal rehabilitation approach, including education, exercises, and bracing, has been proven to be effective in the management of this condition.

In this case, radiographs of the hands (Figure 16.2) reveal narrowing of the right carpometacarpal (CMC) joint, confirming the presence of CMC osteoarthritis (OA). It is common to observe OA in patients with a history of OA in other joints or a family history of OA. The patient discussed in this chapter has a previous history of OA and a hip replacement.

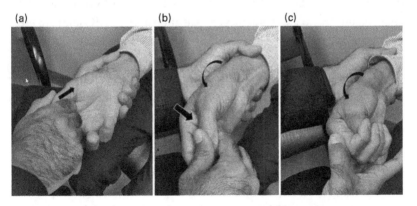

FIGURE 16.1 Physical examination maneuvers for thumb pain. (a) Axial load, (b) Finkelstein's test, (c) Eichhoff's test.

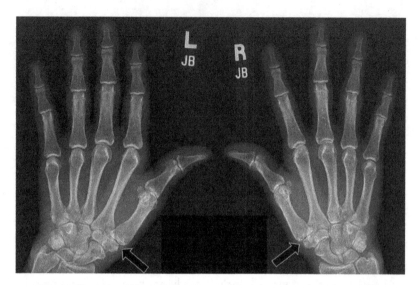

FIGURE 16.2 Bilateral hand X-rays, anteroposterior view. The left (L) hand reveals a normal first carpometacarpal joint, whereas the right (R) side shows narrowing, which is consistent with osteoarthritis.

First CMC OA is a common disease affecting females more than males by a 3:1 ratio. It is usually seen after the fifth decade and can cause pain, laxity, and weakness of handgrip. The pain is caused by degenerative changes of the articulation between the first metacarpal and the trapezium (Figure 16.2) and laxity of the CMC ligaments. Axial load of the CMC joint (Figure 16.1a) and tenderness to palpation at the CMC joint are used as diagnostic clues for this disorder, but the diagnosis of CMC OA is confirmed by plain films or arthroscopy.

The clinical consensus for the treatment of CMC OA is conservative care prior to surgical interventions. CMC OA is treated initially with relative rest (partial immobilization), hand therapy, and corticosteroid injections. Recent studies have demonstrated that 85% of patients with CMC OA have significant clinical improvement of their pain and functional improvements with orthoses (bracing) and hand therapy. Therapy generally consists of exercises for optimizing thumb positioning, stability, range of motion, and improving strength. In patients who require injections, it appears that image-guided injections are not superior to anatomically guided or "blind" injections because neither translates into significant delays in eventual need for surgery. For patients who fail to respond to conservative care, multiple surgical interventions are available, including osteotomies, ligament reconstruction, and joint replacements.

KEY POINTS TO REMEMBER

- De Quervain's tenosynovitis and CMC OA are common causes of pain at the base of the thumb and radial wrist; these are more common in females than males.
- De Quervain tenosynovitis is a tendinosis of the first dorsal wrist compartment, and Finkelstein's and Eichhoff's tests are useful, simple examination maneuvers to help make the diagnosis.
- CMC OA is suspected by tenderness at the CMC joint and axial load of the joint.
- Definite diagnosis of CMC OA is made by radiography or arthroscopy.
- For both diagnoses, orthoses, rehabilitation, and injections are considered effective as initial treatment. In cases that fail conservative management, surgical management may be necessary.
- If untreated, these conditions can result in significant loss of grip strength and disability.

Further Reading

Cavaleri R, Schabrun SM, Te M, et al. Hand therapy versus corticosteroid injections in the treatment of de Quervain's disease: A systematic review and meta-analysis. *J Hand Ther*. 2016;29(1):3–11.

Gershkovich GE, Boyadjian H, Conti Mica M. The effect of image-guided corticosteroid injections on thumb carpometacarpal arthritis. *Hand*. 2019 [Epub ahead of print].

Tsehaie J, Spekreijse KR, Wouters RM, et al. Outcome of a hand orthosis and hand therapy for carpometacarpal osteoarthritis in daily practice: A prospective cohort study. *J Hand Surg Am*. 2018;43(11):1000–1009.

Wu F, Rajpura A, Sandher D. Finkelstein's test is superior to Eichhoff's test in the investigation of de Quervain's disease. *J Hand Microsurg*. 2018;10(2):116–118.

17 Can't Open Jars Due to Crooked Fingers

Bruno Subbarao

A 67-year-old female with a past medical history of rheumatoid arthritis (RA) presents to your office with complaints of pain in her hands, specifically in the joints of her fingers and wrists. The pain is reported worse in the morning and is often accompanied by stiffness and swelling. She has been noncompliant with her medication due to cost. Now her hands appear deformed, and she requests help to decrease pain and improve the function of her hands.

On examination, moderate swelling is noted at the wrists and metacarpophalangeal (MCP) and proximal interphalangeal (PIP) joints of her fingers bilaterally. There is tenderness and warmth to the touch in the affected joints. There is moderate ulnar deviation of the fingers at the MCP joints. In addition, you notice hyperflexion of the PIP joints, with extension at the distal interphalangeal (DIP) joints on her index fingers bilaterally.

What do you do now?

- Rheumatoid arthritis
- Osteoarthritis
- Other systemic condition affecting the hands

Rheumatoid arthritis is a chronic, inflammatory, autoimmune condition that can carry systemic complications but will primarily affect the synovial joints, leading to disability if left untreated. The synovium (joint lining that helps lubricate the joints) is particularly affected in RA. It is common to see inflammation (swelling and warmth) as described in this patient (Figure 17.1). With time, the swelling and inflammation can lead to hypertrophy of the synovium and new tissue growth known as "pannus" formation that

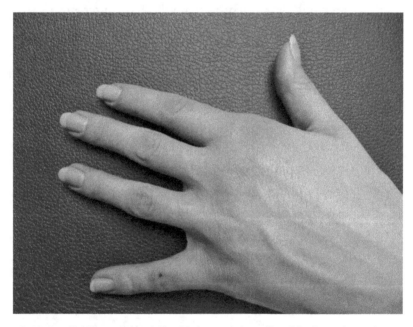

FIGURE 17.1 Early rheumatoid arthritis with characteristic swelling of the first and second metacarpophalangeal joints.

Reprinted with permission from Aletaha, Daniel, and Helga Radner. "Rheumatoid Arthritis—Diagnosis." *Oxford Textbook of Rheumatology*, edited by Richard A. Watts et al. Oxford University Press, 2013.

can stiffen joints. Eventually, this may lead to damage of the articular cartilage and bone and could even cause stretch or rupture of ligaments and tendons, thus leading to instability and deformity.

Differential diagnosis in this patient would include osteoarthritis (OA). In OA, however, we would expect primary involvement of the DIP joints as opposed to the PIP and MCP joints (Figure 17.2). In addition, RA presents more commonly with morning stiffness, and OA would typically be associated with stiffness late in the day after use of the affected joints. An X-ray may help better distinguish the two conditions because OA would not cause the bony erosions we would expect to see in RA and the pattern of joint narrowing would tend to be symmetric in RA as opposed to being seen predominantly on weight-bearing surfaces, a pattern linked to OA.

Other conditions to consider are tendonitis in the hand or forearm and carpal tunnel syndrome. Both would help explain pain and loss of function but would not explain the deformities. However, it is important to keep in mind that with RA there is an increased risk of developing both of these conditions. In fact, one should be very wary of concomitant pathologies with a systemic, autoimmune illness such as RA; these include fatigue, weight loss, osteopenia, vasculitis, uveitis, pleuritis, myocarditis, anemia, and glomerulonephritis.

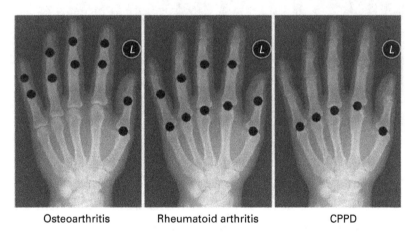

Osteoarthritis   Rheumatoid arthritis   CPPD

FIGURE 17.2 Most common joints affected by arthritic conditions. CPPD, calcium pyrophosphate dehydrate (a crystal arthropathy).

Reprinted with permission from O'Connor, Philip. "Investigating Hand and Wrist Problems." *Musculoskeletal Imaging*, edited by Philip G. Conaghan et al. Oxford University Press, 2010.

This case illustrates some of the unfortunate consequences of long-standing, poorly managed RA. Her history of morning stiffness along with her physical examination yield classic signs of the condition, including the symmetrical swelling, tenderness, and warmth of the hand joints. The MCP and PIP joints are preferentially affected over the DIP joints, and we would expect a loss of range of motion as a result. The ulnar deviation of the fingers at the MCP joints is common as a result of an imbalance of forces on the joints in the set-ting of weakened ligaments and altered biomechanics. The hyperflexion of the PIP joints with extension of the DIP joints observed in the index fingers of this patient is known as Boutonniere's deformity, commonly seen in patients as a chronic effect of RA after damage to the collateral ligaments at the PIP joints. Other types of deformities can occur depending on which joints and ligaments are affected. A swan neck deformity occurs when there is hyperextension of the PIP joint with flexion of the DIP joint (Figure 17.3).

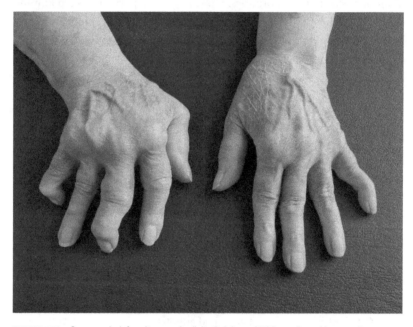

FIGURE 17.3 Swan neck deformity seen in digits 3 right and 5 bilaterally and boutonnière deformity seen in digit 2 of the right hand.

Reprinted with permission from Aletaha, Daniel, and Helga Radner. "Rheumatoid Arthritis—Diagnosis." *Oxford Textbook of Rheumatology*, edited by Richard A. Watts et al. Oxford University Press, 2013.

At this point, plain radiographs of the hands would be warranted to assess for narrowing of the joint spaces, which occurs due to the gradual destruction of the articular cartilage. It is also important to assess for bony erosions on plain films, especially because erosions of the bones are associated with premature mortality, decreased quality of life, and increased risk of disability (Figures 17.4 and 17.5).

Among the first recommendations for this patient would be to follow the advice of her rheumatologist, including the importance of taking recommended anti-rheumatic medications. Disease-modifying antirheumatic drugs (DMARDs) could help prevent or minimize further damage by altering the course of the disease. Cost was raised as an issue contributing to her noncompliance, and she should openly discuss this with her rheumatologist to seek affordable alternatives or programs that may help her afford her medications. This is extremely important given the potential systemic effects of this condition. But cost should always be kept in mind, regardless of the presenting complaint.

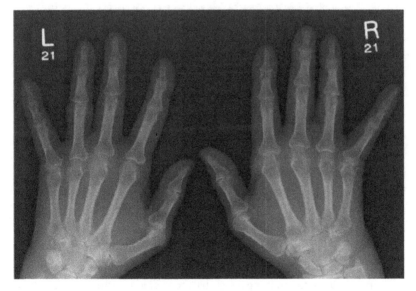

FIGURE 17.4 Hand X-rays of a patient with rheumatoid arthritis demonstrating marked joint space narrowing and osteopenia affecting the MCP joints.

Reprinted with permission from O'Connor, Philip. "Investigating Hand and Wrist Problems." *Musculoskeletal Imaging*, edited by Philip G. Conaghan et al. Oxford University Press, 2010.

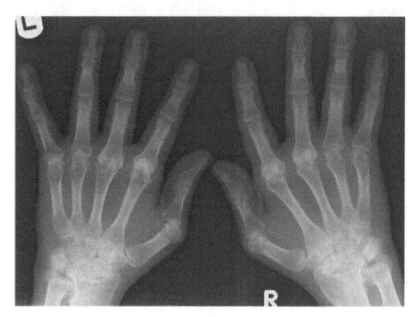

FIGURE 17.5 Bilateral symmetrical arthropathy from rheumatoid arthritis demonstrating bony erosions over the left and right index, middle, and little MCP and right ring MCP joints. Ulnar deviation can be seen affecting the right MCP joints, and erosive changes are present over the carpal bones and radioulnar joints bilaterally.

Reprinted with permission from O'Connor, Philip. "Investigating Hand and Wrist Problems." *Musculoskeletal Imaging*, edited by Philip G. Conaghan et al. Oxford University Press, 2010.

Pain control can be quite challenging in this population due to the complex nature of the condition and the potential that these patients may be on several other medications, increasing the potential for medication interactions and systemic toxicity. The use of a multimodal approach to include nonpharmacological and pharmacological options, psychological treatments, physical therapy modalities, and consideration of surgery when indicated may best optimize care and limit complications.

You should begin with the basics. Educate your patient on living a healthy lifestyle to include smoking cessation if the patient is a smoker and the importance of maintaining a well-balanced diet, routine exercise habits, a proper sleep schedule, and compliance with rheumatological medications.

Next, taking a conservative approach, you can explore nonpharmacological options for pain relief. Nonpharmacological options are plentiful but are limited by availability, costs, and often lack robust scientific evidence. However, because of their benign nature, they may warrant consideration. One example is compression gloves, which are touted to improve hand function and relieve pain. The compression may help prevent swelling and provide warmth, thereby reducing stiffness and potentially improving grip. Other options include splinting of the wrists, hands, or fingers. For example, ring splints can provide comfort and are available to help correct or offset Boutonniere or swan neck deformities or counteract ulnar deviation by supporting the fingers at the MCP joints.

A referral to see an occupational therapist (OT) would not only help find the correct orthoses but also help address loss of functionality. An OT will provide gentle and safe strengthening exercises for the hands as well as stretching techniques to reduce stiffness and maximize functional range of motion. In addition, an OT can provide instructions regarding joint conservation measures and specific modalities under supervision such as paraffin baths, other forms of therapeutic heat/cold, or electrical stimulation to help relieve pain and swelling. Depending on the patient's individual needs, assessment for durable medical equipment can be made to ensure she can keep up with her activities of daily living.

Moving beyond therapies and braces, pharmacological options can potentially provide immediate benefits by reducing pain and inflammation. Of course, it is important to remember that choice of medicine is dependent on multiple factors, including patient willingness, history of compliance with medications, and potential interactions with DMARDs or other medications that the patient may be using. However, two classes of medications are worth considering: nonsteroidal anti-inflammatory drugs and glucocorticoids. Glucocorticoids have the added flexibility of localized or systemic administration through injection or oral administration, respectively.

Once the patient's acute and subacute needs have been addressed, it is critical to discuss long-term management. Specifically, referral to a psychologist is warranted because RA is a lifelong condition associated with pain and disability. Treatment with cognitive–behavioral therapy, a specific type of psychotherapy aimed at developing or improving coping strategies and changing the way pain is thought about or viewed, has demonstrated modest improvements in pain and disability for RA patients. Mindfulness training, a strategy in which focus is taken away from pain and placed elsewhere on tasks, self, or the environment at the moment, may also be a valuable option depending on availability.

Last, referral to a hand surgeon may be needed depending on the level of pain, functional disability, and extent of hand deformities present. Surgical procedures are numerous and can include arthrodesis, tendon realignment, synovectomy, and other reconstructive surgeries. These surgeries carry some potential risks, but if implemented in a timely manner, may have the ability to improve function, reduce pain, reduce deformity, and slow disease progression.

KEY POINTS TO REMEMBER

- Rheumatoid arthritis is a chronic, inflammatory, autoimmune condition that characteristically affects the joints, commonly starting with the hands and feet, in a symmetric manner.
- Pain is most effectively managed through a multimodal approach utilizing pharmaceuticals, physical modalities, and psychological interventions.
- Consultation with a rheumatologist as soon as possible is essential for management of RA.
- Imaging can assess and qualify the extent of injury to the joints and help with prognosis.

Further Reading

Burmester GR, Pope JE. Novel treatment strategies in rheumatoid arthritis. *Lancet.* 2017;389(10086):2338–2348. doi:10.1016/s0140-6736(17)31491-5

Rubin DA. MRI and ultrasound of the hands and wrists in rheumatoid arthritis: I. Imaging findings. *Skeletal Radiol.* 2019;48(5):677–695. doi:10.1007/s00256-019-03179-z

Walsh DA, Mcwilliams DF. Mechanisms, impact and management of pain in rheumatoid arthritis. *Nature Rev Rheumatol.* 2014;10(10):581–592. doi:10.1038/nrrheum.2014.64

18 A Locking Ring Finger

Ramon Cuevas-Trisan

A 58-year-old male complains of pain in the right hand associated with locking of the ring finger for the past 4 or 5 months. He denies any redness or trauma to the hand but states that the hand has swollen occasionally. His past medical history is remarkable for type 2 diabetes mellitus, hypertension, and mild obesity.

On inspection, the hands appear remarkable for callous formation over the palmar surface along several metacarpophalangeal (MCP) joints. There are no open wounds and there are no signs of inflammation. Sensation is normal and he is able to make a strong fist bilaterally without limitations in range of motion. There is slight tenderness at the base of the right ring finger (over the area of the MCP joint). When you ask him to actively make a fist and open the hand while you palpate the tender area, you detect a slight snapping and feel a small nodule.

What do you do now?

- Trigger finger
- Dupuytren's disease
- Diabetic cheiroarthropathy
- Metacarpophalangeal joint sprain or arthritis
- Non-infectious tenosynovitis

The patient presents with fairly localized discrete pain in the hand. Pain is over the ring finger MCP joint, and there are no signs of trauma or infection. The patient is diabetic, raising the concern for a commonly unrecognized condition known as diabetic cheiroarthropathy. The condition is caused by a generalized thickening of the skin that leads to contractures of the fingers that may be seen in nearly one-third of patients with long-standing diabetes mellitus (type 1 more frequently than type 2). The fingers may appear edematous with thick, tight, and waxy skin. Affected individuals may develop flexion contractures with inability to fully extend the finger joints (inability to place hands fully flat on a surface). However, this condition tends to affect both hands and multiple joints as opposed to causing a localized contracture. The condition is usually painless, but numbness and pain may be experienced with concomitant neuropathy or microvascular disease of the hand. Management includes stretching exercises and tight blood glucose control.

Another possibility would be the early stages of Dupuytren's disease. This a relatively common disorder in which the palmar fascia progressively fibroses leading to stiffness and eventual finger flexion contractures over months to years. Histologically, there is palmar fascial thickening (fibroblast proliferation with dense collagen that does not infiltrate deeper tissues) as part of a benign, yet potentially disabling, fibroproliferative process. Its etiology is unknown, but some demographic factors that are commonly observed are male gender, generally older than age 50 years, and more commonly in whites. Diabetes, cigarette smoking, and alcohol use are also considered risk factors. Its relationship to use of vibration tools and repetitive handling tasks has been suggested but not decisively proven.

Dupuytren's disease is usually painless but at times, particularly in its early stages, may present as palpable nodules that may be tender. Pain may also be present when there is a concomitant tenosynovitis. The condition tends to predominantly affect the fourth and fifth fingers, with the index and thumb rarely involved. The first symptom reported is thickening or a bump in the palm around the flexor crease of the affected finger(s).Diagnosis is based on the history and physical examination findings. Imaging studies are not needed nor contributory because there is no calcification of the tendons or surrounding soft tissues. On examination, there are typically no signs of inflammation. Initially there may just be a palpable nodule over the flexor tendon in the distal part of the palm. Over time, this progresses to palpable fibrous cords that cause puckering of the skin, limiting finger extension (at the MCP and proximal interphalangeal joints), eventually causing irreversible flexion contractures of these joints (Figure 18.1). This condition

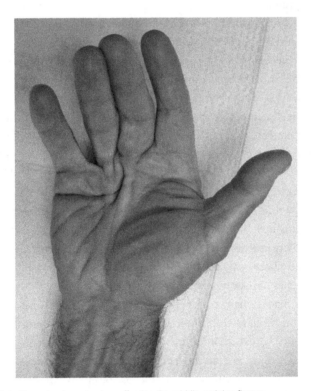

FIGURE 18.1 Dupuytren's contracture affecting the middle and ring fingers.

must also be distinguished from malignant lesions such as epithelioid sarcomas, which are more common in teenagers and young adults, sometimes presenting as palmar fibromatosis and ulcerations.

Management of Dupuytren's disease depends on the stage and severity of the condition. In its early stages, use of padded gloves and cushioned handles for occupational tasks tend to be beneficial. Splinting and exercise are sometimes used, but there is lack of scientific evidence for their effectiveness in preventing contracture progression. In fact, there are concerns about stretching potentially worsening the condition, based on upregulation of fibroblasts when tension is applied, seen in laboratory studies. Corticosteroid injections are sometimes used, particularly when there is local tenderness. Some studies have shown regression of nodules, but more often long-term results are disappointing. In addition, these injections may lead to complications including skin atrophy, infection, and tendon rupture.

Management of contractures as the disease progresses generally requires surgical interventions but in select cases may respond to collagenase *Clostridium histolyticum* injections. Collagenases are proteinases that hydrolyze collagen in its native triple-helical conformation under physiological conditions, resulting in lysis of collagen deposits. These injections are sometimes tried earlier in the disease when contractures are not very severe (less than 40–50 degrees) in patients who opt for nonsurgical management. These injections are performed as an office-based procedure followed by manipulation (passive finger extension) by the provider 24–72 hours after the injections. These may be repeated every 4 weeks up to three times per site. Side effects are common but generally mild (injection site pain, ecchymosis, and edema), but serious adverse events include tendon rupture, ligament damage, nerve injury, and hypersensitivity reactions. Short-term efficacy has been generally described as highly beneficial, particularly for less severe contractures, but long-term recurrence rates have been reported to be close to 50%.

Surgical management is generally necessary as the disease progresses. Techniques include fasciectomy (excision of fascial cords) and fasciotomy (transection of cords) in order to improve hand function by correction of contractures. Recurrence rates are generally higher in younger patients. A less invasive procedure (percutaneous needle fasciotomy or aponeurectomy) is sometimes used but has a high recurrence rate.

The patient in this case appears to be suffering from a trigger finger (stenosing flexor tenosynovitis). This condition may be confused with early Dupuytren's disease, but the finger flexion "contracture" of a trigger finger is a dynamic one that is corrected as opposed to the one created by Dupuytren's disease. Trigger finger is one of the most common painful hand conditions in adults, generally in the 50- to 70-year-old range. It is more common in females and has a higher prevalence in patients with diabetes and rheumatoid arthritis. The condition tends to be idiopathic, although it has sometimes been attributed to hand overuse.

Patients with this condition describe catching or snapping of the affected finger during active flexion and extension. There may be impairment of voluntary extension often requiring passive manipulation with the other hand to extend the finger. The catching or snapping may be painful, with pain sometimes radiating from the MCP area distally into the finger(s).

Tendon sheaths of the long flexors run from the level of the meta-carpal heads to the distal phalanges. They are attached to the underlying bones and volar plates, which prevent the tendons from bowstringing. Thickenings in the fibrous flexor sheath act as pulleys, directing the sliding movements of the fingers. The two types of pulleys are annular (A) and cruciate (C). Annular pulleys are composed of single fibrous bands, whereas cruciate pulleys have two crossing fibrous bands. The A1 pulley overlies the MCP joints and is by far the most commonly involved pulley in trigger finger, although cases of triggering have been reported at the second and third annular pulleys (A2 and A3), as well as the palmar aponeurosis. The pathophysiology of this condition has generally been described as patho-logical changes at the pulley. However, direct intraoperative observation of the affected tendons has shown changes in their appearance resembling those seen in tendons affected by tendinosis (also observed in the tendons histologically). It has thus been postulated that repeated friction and com-pression between the flexor tendon and the corresponding inner layer of the A1 pulley results in fibrocartilagenous metaplasia, causing local thickening. Inflammation and hypertrophy of the retinacular sheath progressively re-strict the motion of the flexor tendon, causing the tendon to get stuck at the proximal edge of the A1 pulley when the patient is attempting to extend the digit. The end result is thickening (or nodules) of the pulley, flexor tendon or sheaths that disrupts the normal gliding motion under the tendon under the pulley as the finger flexes and extends (Figure 18.2). In severe cases, the finger may become locked in flexion or extension, requiring passive manipulation of the finger to fully flex or extend.

Imaging studies are not necessary in diagnosing a patient with suspected trigger finger. The diagnosis is based on a history of locking or clicking during finger movement. The patient is asked to hold the hand in the palms-up position and asked to actively flex and extend the fingers to try to make the finger lock or catch. In milder cases, when triggering is not readily observed, the clinician can palpate the MCP joint as the finger is actively flexed and extended, noting the presence of loss of smooth motion or a clicking sensation (as in this case). Pain or tenderness directly over the tendon as it courses over the MCP joint is sometimes present. The presence of multiple trigger fingers is not uncommon.

Management of trigger finger involves conservative and invasive options. In the early stages, activity modification, splinting, and/or short-term nonsteroidal anti-inflammatory drugs may be useful. Activity modification consists of avoiding potentially aggravating movements such as pinching or grasping of the fingers. Splinting involves immobilization of the MCP joint with a metal finger splint or a custom thermoplastic splint. The splint should keep the MCP joint in slight flexion and can be worn based on trigger pattern and patient preferences (daytime, nighttime, or with activity). The splint should generally be worn for 3–6 weeks. A local corticosteroid injection may be offered to patients whose symptoms have not resolved with conservative management. The efficacy of corticosteroid injections has been demonstrated in many observational studies. The injection may be

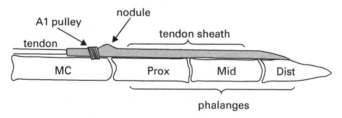

FIGURE 18.2 Diagram of anatomic structures involved in trigger finger. Note that this is a pictorial representation of one of the theories of the pathophysiology; local thickening of the pulley is another proposed mechanism. Dist, distal; MC, metacarpal; Mid, middle; Prox, proximal.

repeated in 4–6 weeks if symptoms have not improved, but most patients experience significant improvement with a single injection. Adverse effects from corticosteroid injections for trigger finger are rare but include atrophy of the subcutaneous fat, tendon rupture, and hypopigmentation.

Surgical release is generally reserved for patients who have failed conservative therapy and have not improved with corticosteroid injections. Percutaneous and open surgical releases of the A1 pulley are both effective, with very low recurrence rates. Complications from the procedures include infection, nerve injury, flexor tendon bowstringing (protrusion of the flexor tendon into the palm with finger flexion), and tendon scarring. Outcomes of surgery may not be as successful in diabetics, who also tend to have higher rates of complications such as infections and need for surgical revisions.

KEY POINTS TO REMEMBER

- Trigger finger is one of the most common adult hand painful conditions.
- Trigger finger may cause a finger flexion "contracture" that is dynamic and corrected versus Dupuytren's disease that causes a true flexion contracture that cannot be manually corrected.
- Conditions to consider in a diabetic patient with finger flexion "contractures" include trigger finger, Dupuytren's disease, and diabetic cheiroarthropathy.
- Trigger fingers and Dupuytren's contractures tend to be more isolated or localized, in contrast to diabetic chieroarthropathy, which causes more generalized finger contractures.
- Conservative care tends to be beneficial for trigger finger but less so for Dupuytren's disease. Both conditions may require invasive and surgical management for correction.

Further Reading
Ball C, Izadi D, Verjee LS, Chan J, Nanchahal J. Systematic review of non-surgical treatments for early Dupuytren's disease. *BMC Musculoskelet Disord.* 2016;17(1):345–362.

Fiorini HJ, Tamaoki MJ, Lenza M, et al. Surgery for trigger finger. *Cochrane Database Syst Rev.* 2018;2018(2):CD009860.

Makkouk AH, Oetgen ME, Swigart CR, Dodd SD. Trigger finger: Etiology, evaluation, and treatment. *Curr Rev Musculoskelet Med.* 2008;1:92–96.

McAuliffe JA. Tendon disorders of the hand and wrist. *J Hand Surg.* 2010;35(5):846–853.

Peters-Veluthamaningal C, van der Windt DA, Winters JC, Meyboom-de Jong B. Corticosteroid injection for trigger finger in adults. *Cochrane Database Syst Rev.* 2009;2009(2):CD005617.

Townley WA, Baker R, Sheppard N, Grobbelaar AO. Dupuytren's contracture unfolded. *BMJ.* 2006;332:397–400.

Trojian TH, Chu SM. Dupuytren's disease: Diagnosis and treatment. *Am Fam Physician.* 2007;76(1):86–89.

19 Ghostly White Hands That Come and Go

Maricarmen Cruz-Jimenez and Ramon Cuevas-Trisan

A 27-year-old female complains about episodic hand discoloration and pain in the fingers for the past 6–8 weeks that seems to be getting progressively worse. She describes that her fingers get very pale for 15–30 minutes followed by turning beefy red, throbbing, and swelling. Medical history is significant for occasional knee swelling but is otherwise unremarkable. She uses no medications except birth control pills.

Her hands have normal color but the tips of her left middle and index fingers are very dry and slightly pitted. Ulnar and radial pulses are normal but capillary refill in all fingers (except the thumbs) is very sluggish. Some of her metacarpophalangeal and proximal interphalangeal joints are tender to palpation. Hand sensation appears to be intact. Grip strength is good, but she reports some pain at some of metacarpophalangeal joints when gripping. Her knees appear slightly swollen and warm to the touch.

What do you do now?

- Does the patient have a systemic problem causing all her symptoms?
- Is there a vascular problem possibly causing intermittent circulatory impairment to the hands?
- What additional physical examination tests could be performed in order to formulate a presumptive diagnosis?
- Should any imaging or laboratory tests be ordered to better evaluate this patient?

This patient presents with a couple of complaints that may or may not be related. Her chief complaint is suggestive of a vascular problem but her pulses are normal. The description of the episodic discoloration and painful bouts of her fingers suggest the possibility that this is a Raynaud's phenomenon. The clinician can perform a simple test in the office: the patient could be asked to immerse her hands in cold water to determine if exposure to cold temperature triggers one such episode. This test is done, and it triggers the symptoms that she had described.

In evaluating the patient's history, her secondary complaints, and physical examination findings, it becomes evident that the patient may be suffering from an underlying connective tissue disorder and that the Raynaud's seen in her case could be secondary to such disorder. The pattern of joint complaints and findings on examination suggest the possible presence of rheumatoid arthritis. Therefore, imaging studies and laboratory tests [rheumatoid factor, erythrocyte sedimentation rate (ESR), anti-nuclear antibody (ANA), etc.] along with a referral to a rheumatologist appear to be in order.

Raynaud's is a rare condition that impacts approximately 5% of the U.S. population. This condition affects arteries, particularly at their most distal segments of the fingers and to a lesser degree the toes. The vessels suffer severe vasospasm that leads to ischemia and pain (Figure 19.1). The pathophysiology is not clearly understood, and although most of the evidence suggests that peripheral mechanisms are considered responsible for the symptoms, some evidence suggests that there may be central mechanisms contributing to the pathophysiology due to the eventual

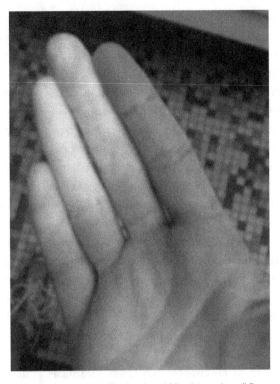

FIGURE 19.1 Raynaud's phenomenon affecting the middle, ring, and small fingers.

manifestation of internal organ damage. The condition is described as primary or secondary. Its primary form is sometimes referred to as Raynaud's disease. Its cause is unknown (idiopathic), and it is more common and tends to be less severe than secondary Raynaud's. Its secondary form, called Raynaud's phenomenon, is seen as part of other systemic underlying conditions. Such conditions may include rheumatological diseases (connective tissue disorders including scleroderma and systemic lupus erythematosus), smoking, hand trauma (including use of vibration tools), extrinsic vascular obstruction, paraproteinemias and certain drugs/chemicals such as β-blockers, contraceptive medications, vinyl chloride, and mercury exposure. Cold temperatures and emotional stress trigger the vasospasm sensory symptoms (including paresthesias, numbness, and severe pain) and dramatic changes in the appearance of the affected area. During an attack, the affected areas initially turn pale. Then, they often turn cyanotic and feel cold and numb. As the area warms up and circulation is restored, the area may swell and turn red. This is usually accompanied by throbbing and tingling. In severe cases, ulceration and gangrene may be seen.

Risk factors vary between the primary and secondary Raynaud's. In primary disease, risk factors include gender (female preponderance), age younger than 30 years, family history, and living in cold climates. In Raynaud's phenomenon, risk factors include age older than 30 years, diseases that directly damage arteries or nerves that supply those arteries, injuries to hands and feet, exposure to certain chemicals, repetitive activities of the hand, smoking, cold climate, and exposure to some medications.

The diagnosis is made by triggering the vasospasm using tests such as the cold stimulation test. The assessment consists of placing the hand in cold water with a device that measures temperature. Patients with Raynaud's will require more than 20 minutes to return to their normal temperature. Other workup should be completed seeking underlying conditions related to secondary Raynaud's; these tests include ANA, ESR, and C-reactive protein blood tests, among others.

Because there is no cure for Raynaud's, treatment goals are centered on patient education, their awareness on how to protect their hands from attacks, and lifestyle modifications. This will be done through the combination of patient education, avoiding cold temperatures, and wearing gloves. Patients should seek ways to manage their stress, avoid vibrating equipment, and avoid repetitive hand activities. Other lifestyle changes to consider are smoking cessation and limiting the consumption of caffeine and alcohol. Triggering medications such as β-blockers, migraine medications containing ergotamine, and birth control pills should be avoided.

Some medications can alleviate symptoms; these include calcium channel blockers (nifedipine and amlodipine being first-line agents), topical nitrates, and α-blockers. Calcium channel blockers, in particular, have the ability to improve the frequency, duration, and severity of attacks and can also improve its associated pain and disability. In severe cases, and particularly when skin ulcerations persist, sympathetic blocks (stellate ganglion/lumbar sympathetic) may provide longer relief by increasing circulation and decreasing pain. There is increasing but limited evidence to support the use of type A botulinum toxin in the management of Raynaud's phenomenon. Small case series have been reported showing significant improvement in perfusion to the digits. This treatment is usually considered when multiple other modalities of treatment have failed and has been reported to heal recalcitrant digit ulcers leading to prevention of amputations. One of the authors has had some experience in a small number of patients with excellent results. The mechanism of action is unknown but is theorized to possibly induce relaxation of the arteriole vasculature, thus improving perfusion.

The quality of life (QOL) of patients who suffer from Raynaud's is significantly affected, both their psychological well-being and their physical functioning. In secondary Raynaud's, other factors can impact functional independence and QOL, including disabling pain, contractures, ulcers, and amputations. Although lifestyle modification lead to vasospasm attack prevention, 64% of patients report having a poor ability to prevent them. Providers should work on revisiting goals of care with regularity so that timely interventions are addressed, including psychological support, palliative measures, orthotic equipment, and energy conservation techniques. In this case, in addition to investigating the presence of a connective tissue disorder and starting appropriate management, the patient should be educated about avoiding triggers such as exposure to cold, consider another type of contraception method, and exercise caution to avoid exposure to toxic chemicals.

KEY POINTS TO REMEMBER

- Raynaud's is a vascular condition that may be idiopathic (primary) or a manifestation of a systemic disease (secondary).
- Secondary Raynaud's is primarily managed by treating the underlying cause and avoiding triggers.
- Raynaud's can be very disabling and painful, leading to finger and toe amputations in extreme/severe cases.

Further Reading

Hughes M, Snapir A, Wilkinson J, Snapir D, Wigley FM, Herrick AL. Prediction and impact of attacks of Raynaud's phenomenon, as judged by patient perception.

Rheumatology. 2015;54(8):1443–1447. https://doi.org/10.1093/rheumatology/kev002

National Heart, Lung, and Blood Institute. *Raynaud's.* Retrieved December 7, 2019, from https://www.nhlbi.nih.gov/health-topics/raynauds

Rirash F, Tingey PC, Hardin SE, et al. Calcium channel blockers for primary and secondary Raynaud's phenomenon. *Cochrane Database Syst Rev.* 2017;2017(12): CD000467. doi:10.1002/14651858.CD000467.pub2

Żebryk P, Puszczewicz MJ. Botulinum toxin A in the treatment of Raynaud's phenomenon: A systematic review. *Arch Med Sci.* 2016;12(4):864–870. doi:10.5114/aoms.2015.48152

Very Bothersome
Ballooning Arm

Keryl Motta-Valencia and
Ady M. Correa-Mendoza

A 67-year-old female complains of left arm pain and
limited motion during the past several weeks. Pain
is diffuse, sometimes lancinating, associated with
swelling of the arm. Symptoms have progressed,
becoming constant and interfering with all activities.
She denies recent trauma or any skin wounds.
Physical examination shows mild erythema and
pitting edema (+2), worse distally. Distal pulses
feel weak but capillary refill is 2 seconds with no
cyanosis. There is allodynia on the arm, joints are
nontender, but overall arm motion and strength are
limited by pain inhibition. Spurling's test is negative
with no upper motor neuron signs.

Review of systems is remarkable for low-grade
fever. Her medical history is remarkable for metabolic
syndrome and left breast fibroadenoma, status
post lumpectomy (30 years prior). Family history
is remarkable for breast cancer (mother and sister,
both prior to age 50 years). Her childhood history
includes bilateral lower extremities lymphedema that
developed at age 8 years (undetermined cause).

What do you do now?

DISCUSSION QUESTIONS

- What could be causing the patient's subacute and painful left upper extremity limb swelling that has adversely affected her quality of life and function in recent weeks? Could this be a neurological problem?
- Could the swelling be linked to an underlying medical condition? Consideration should also be given to intrinsic patient risk factors for breast cancer, along with a strong family history (risk is doubled by one first-degree relative, escalating to five times higher than average risk for two first-line relatives). Yet, she has preexistent congenital lymphedema, so is she presenting an evolution of a preexistent disorder or are new medical conditions involved?

The patient's disabling left arm presentation of severe diffuse pain and swelling over a relatively rapid time frame despite no identified trauma or trigger events warrants a thorough and comprehensive evaluation. A critical analysis of the patient's symptoms and signs will be helpful in narrowing the differential diagnosis. Descriptors about her pain are valuable in assessing her clinical presentation. She complained of allodynia (tingling), which does not necessarily indicate a neural injury but suggests sensitization. Her neuropathic-type pain (numbness, heaviness, and lancinating) may be associated with radicular, brachial plexus, and/or focal nerve entrapment injuries. If physical examination had demonstrated signs of hyperpathia and dysesthesia, it could hint about a complex regional pain syndrome (type 1 or 2), especially if associated with dystrophic and vasomotor changes of skin and its appendages.

Visual inspection of skin is important to detect wounds or portals of entry, as expected for cellulitis or infectious processes. Examination should also seek masses, lumps, and/or deformities. A fracture is unexpected for her nontraumatic history, the exception being pathologic fractures that may debut spontaneously with diffuse pain, swelling, and limitation in motion. A compartment syndrome of the upper limb is rare and would likely be seen in the setting of trauma, exertional, or cumulative repetitive stress exposures.

The clinical assessment of the patient's vascular system is suggestive of patent arterial branches and veins; however, there may be problems with lymphatic drainage. In contrast to her primary leg lymphedema that usually features nonpitting edema, her newly acquired limb swelling is characterized by pitting edema and involves a different anatomic region. Therefore, her differential diagnosis encompasses primary and acquired causes for a secondary lymphedema, which in the context of the upper limb include various potential etiologies, summarized in Table 20.1.

TABLE 20.1 **Etiologies per Lymphedema Category**

Category	Specific Features
Primary lymphedema	
Congenital lymphedema	Lymphangioma (birth−2 years)
Lymphedema praecox	Before age 35 years
Lymphedema tarda	After age 35 years
Hereditary lymphedema	Genetic mutations: *GJC2, FOXC2, CCBE1, VGFR-3, PTPN14, GATA2,* and *SOX18*
Lymphangioma	Rare, cystic, benign growth
Secondary lymphedema	

Systemic causes	Inflammatory: chronic onset, progressive
	   Infection (cellulitis)
	   Lipedema
	   Rheumatic disease
	Cardiac insufficiency
	Renal disease

Vascular	Chronic venous insufficiency
Metabolic	Thyroid disease Diabetes mellitus Hypoalbuminemia

Musculoskeletal	Tendinopathy
	Bony lesions
	Compartment syndrome
	Fractures
	   Traumatic
	   Pathologic

Continued

TABLE 20.1 **Continued**

Category	Specific Features
Neurologic	Complex regional pain syndrome

Malignancies: associated with weight loss, fatigue, pain, nerve lesions	Skin (melanoma)
	Head and neck
	Genitourinary (bladder, prostate)
	Primary sarcomas of the extremities
	Gynecological (cervix, ovary)
	Gynecological (breast cancer-related)
	Neuropathy
	    Axillary web syndrome
	    Chemotherapy-induced neuropathy
	    Mastectomy-related thoracic outlet
	    syndrome

The subacute limb swelling and underlying medical factors in this patient warrant further workup, a decision further supported by the accompanying symptoms of mild fever and her individual risk factors. Her medical history is remarkable for advanced age, combined with a breast nodule in the context of a strong family history, raising a flag for the occurrence of a malignant lymphedema due to infiltrative tumors affecting lymph nodes or blocking their drainage. Masses occurring in the thorax or proximal upper limb may compress the thoracic outlet, leading to lymphatic drainage blockage. When a mass infiltrates the lower trunks of the brachial plexus, it is more likely to generate severe pain and might correlate with tissue growth rate, as suspected in the case of this patient. In contrast, involvement at the upper trunk of the brachial plexus is more likely to occur in post-radiation cases and characterized by dull neuropathic pain.

Lymphedema occurs due to accumulation of high-protein fluid at the interstitial tissues when dysfunction or obstructions impair lymph transport along the lymphatic system. Early symptoms include discomfort, heaviness, swelling, and pitting edema. Fluid extravasation facilitates inflammatory and fibrotic changes in the subcutaneous tissues. If left untreated, it tends to progress in staging and severity. Final stages occur as fat hypertrophy infiltrates the interstitial space, leading to clinical features of nonpitting edema, elephantiasis, and tumoral degeneration.

Both primary and secondary lymphedema are mostly seen in the lower limbs. Primary lymphedema accounts for 5–10% of cases and arises from congenital and hereditary causes, including mutations. It has greater prevalence among females and a preference for affecting the lower limbs. It has been associated with genetic syndromes and cutaneous disorders, such as Turner syndrome, Klinefelter syndrome, Noonan syndrome, certain trisomy disorders (21, 13, and 18), neurofibromatosis I, hemangiomas, and xanthomatosis. The leading cause of secondary lymphedema worldwide is filariasis. However, in developed countries, the main cause is cancer and/or its therapies (surgical or radiation). A greater incidence of secondary lymphedema is linked to solid tumors because of their tendency for regional lymphatic metastases, but individual incidence varies according to the associated malignancy (e.g., 16% incidence of upper limb lymphedema in melanomas).

A swollen limb may be the manifestation of underlying medical conditions. Workup should include laboratory testing to assess metabolic function (liver, kidney, and thyroid function) and systemic inflammatory status (erythrocyte sedimentation rate, C-reactive protein, and D-dimers). Imaging may include chest radiographs, cardiovascular studies (electrocardiogram), vascular studies (Doppler ultrasound studies), and advanced anatomic imaging of the affected anatomic region [computed tomography or magnetic resonance imaging (MRI)]. Electrodiagnostic studies (electromyography/nerve conduction studies) can be of value in select cases for identifying and localizing suspected peripheral nerve/plexus lesions. In addition, for personal risk factors or a strong family history of breast cancer, a comprehensive workup following current guideline recommendations would include additional testing, such as tests for abnormal genes (*BRCA1*, *BRCA2*, and *CHEK2*), carcinoembryonic antigen, imaging (mammogram, MRI, or ultrasound of breast), and/or biopsy (ultrasound-guided or open).

Lymphedema assessment with circumferential measures of the limb can be easily obtained in the clinical setting, and data may be extrapolated to volumetric measures. Diagnostic threshold values include an interlimb circumference difference of 2 cm of a single measure or 5 cm for the sum of all measurements. The water displacement method accommodates irregularly shaped limb volumes. A difference of more than 10% between limbs suggests the diagnosis. Devices available for lymphedema assessment include the perometer, which uses optoelectronic sensors and infrared light for volumetric assessment; bioimpedance spectroscopy, which uses tissue impedance to assess the extracellular tissue volume; and tissue tonometry, which measures tissue compressibility to correlate with limb swelling.

Imaging workup for lymphedema is helpful for depicting the anatomical and functional status of the lymphatic system's vessels, nodes, and interstitial space. Radionuclide lymphoscintigraphy (LSG) is the accepted standard to confirm the diagnosis of lymphedema. A technetium-labeled colloid is injected into the skin and nuclear scanning generates serial spot images of the tracer during its course from the hand to the axilla. The study depicts anatomical details of the lymphatic system. Another techniques, indocyanine green lymphography using an infrared camera, provides real-time visualization of superficial (<2-cm skin-deep) lymphatic vessel functioning. It provides useful information in cases in which lymphatic–venous shunt (LVS) surgery is a consideration. Magnetic resonance lymphography provides disease staging and surgical planning; it is particularly useful for reconstructive surgery or alternative surgical approaches [microsurgical reconstruction, liposuction, direct excision (resection), or LVS].

Lymphedema is sometimes classified based on physical findings. Stage 0 refers to a subclinical presentation, in which the patient may refer subjective symptoms in the absence of evident swelling. There is impaired lymph transport with minimal changes in tissues that may persist for months to years before the patient develops changes in limb volumes. In stage 1, there is reversible pitting edema that resolves with limb elevation, representing the accumulation of high-protein fluid in the interstitial space. Stage 2 is manifested by irreversible edema that is no longer pitting because lymphostatic fibrosis and excessive fat accumulation have occurred. In this stage, skin infections may be seen. Stage 3 is the most severe form of lymphedema, manifested as elephantiasis, in which there are extreme variations in limb volumes and trophic changes such as acanthosis or warts.

Nonsurgical treatments are generally considered first. Complete decongestive therapy (CDT) is considered the standard of care, and its multimodality approach consists of manual lymphatic drainage, bandaging, prescribed exercise, and skin care. It is initiated by a reduction phase (phase 1) consisting of intense treatment frequency (five times per week) and elastic bandage applications to achieve progressive volume reduction.

When limb volume stabilizes, the maintenance phase (phase 2) consists of providing lower frequency lymphatic drainage sessions (one to three times per week) and individually fitted compression garments for lifetime wear. CDT should be extended for 3–6 months in stages 0–3 lymphedema prior to considering surgical options.

Surgical procedures would be considered when conservative measures have failed. Traditional surgical approaches focus on resecting damaged interstitial tissues or hypertrophied fat and reconstruction of lymphatic vessels or nodes. Specific surgical techniques are beyond the scope of this chapter, but in general, the main surgical approaches are resection techniques (debulking), liposuction, microsurgical reconstruction, and lymph node transfer (Table 20.2).

Recent surgical techniques have expanded the therapeutic alternatives for early lymphedema, including microsurgical reconstructive techniques, vascularized lymph node transfers, and lipoaspiration. A systematic review showed supportive evidence for the latter, specifically for stage 2 upper limb lymphedema that is no longer attaining edema reduction from prolonged compressive therapy.

TABLE 20.2 **Lymphedema Stages and Treatment**

Stage	Findings	Treatment
0	Impaired lymphatics system without evident swelling	Weight loss Compressive decongestive therapy Microsurgical reconstruction
1	Reversible pitting edema without tissue changes	Microsurgical reconstruction Vascularized lymph node transfer
2	Irreversible nonpitting edema with fibrosis	Vascularized lymph node transfer Debulking surgery
3	End-stage lymphedema, elephantiasis. No pitting edema and the presence of trophic skin changes	Debulking surgery

Note: All treatments will be followed by compressive garments use.

Low-level laser therapy (LLLT), also called photobiomodulation therapy, has been researched and increasingly used during recent years, especially for cases of breast cancer-related lymphedema. This modality utilizes phototherapy at varied wavelengths (650 and 1000 nm) that is absorbed by some components of the mitochondria, leading to chain reactions that result in cell proliferation, stimulation of lymphatic vessels, and enhanced fluid circulation to local tissues. Some effects of this therapy are decreased inflammation, lymph vessel regeneration, and prevention of tissue fibrosis. High-quality evidence demonstrating therapeutic effects of this modality is limited, but some randomized controlled trials have shown short-term reductions in upper limb edema with LLLT compared to no treatment.

The association of lymphedema with obesity and lack of exercise suggests an important role for lifestyle modifications. Favorable outcomes from evidence-based exercise interventions specific to breast-related arm lymphedema support the role of physical activity by means of implementing gradual weight-lifting programs. Participation can be aided by preventive use of sleeves and a circuit style for alternating arm–leg activity with rest pauses.

Treatment delays are considered detrimental because the delicate lymphatic valve will eventually suffer permanent damage. Skin care is crucial for the management and prevention of recurrent lymphedema. Bacterial colonization in a setting of a compromised immune system (as in patients with secondary lymphedema) may predispose patients to recurrent infections and worsening of lymphatic system function. Therefore, daily meticulous skin inspection and hygiene are crucial methods to monitor the condition and reduce bacterial bioburden. Current recommendations are similar to skin therapies used in other conditions such as diabetic stasis and pressure sores due to similarities in the cellular characteristics of chronic nonhealing ulcers. Patients should maintain good nail hygiene to reduce bacterial and fungal entry sites. Also, moisturizing soaps and daily application of emollients are recommended to avoid excessive skin dryness. Topical steroids, antifungals, and antimicrobials may be used for lymphedema-associated conditions and sometimes are required for long-term use. For more severe trophic changes of lymphedema, keratolytic agents and salicylic acid have been used.

Arm swelling and discomfort may be encountered during the year following breast surgery while the body adapts and compensates for resected lymph nodes and vessels. Its differential diagnosis includes peri-scar neuropathy of cutaneous nerves in the regions of axilla, chest, and inside arm; axillary web syndrome arising from a residual painful cord after lymph node removal; chemotherapy-induced neuropathy; and mastectomy-related thoracic outlet syndrome following reconstructive surgery. The incidence of post-mastectomy lymphedema has decreased with the advent of more conservative surgical approaches as opposed to radical mastectomy with removal of all lymph nodes. Modern surgical approaches spare the metastasis-negative lymph nodes and remove only those nodes absolutely necessary for staging and management. A sentinel lymph node biopsy has minimal risk of lymphedema, albeit somewhat greater tendency is attributed for axillary node dissection during surgery. A lifetime precaution for the surgically intervened areas is to avoid deep massage.

Pain in lymphedema has been associated with greater psychiatric burden, higher distress, impaired body image, and decreased sexual drive. Thus, early screening is essential to determine if a patient may benefit from evaluation by a mental health or pain management specialist. Limb pain in lymphedema may also be associated with chronic and less recognized etiologies. Soft tissue pressure and guarding with limited use of the limb induced by lymphedema may lead to myofascial pain syndromes and other musculoskeletal ailments, including bursitis, tendinopathy, and arthritis. Severe/persistent pain warrants other conditions to be ruled out, including recurrence of malignancy causing radiculopathy or myelopathy and superimposed infections. Neuropathic pain complaints should raise suspicion for radiation fibrosis, radiation-induced plexopathy, chemotherapy-induced peripheral neuropathy, or an entrapment neuropathy.

Currently, there is only limited evidence regarding the best pharmacological approaches for treating lymphedema-related pain. The nonsteroidal anti-inflammatory drug (NSAID) ketoprofen is commonly used due to its fast absorption and ability to cross the blood–brain barrier. However, like all NSAIDs, its chronic use is limited by side effects of gastrointestinal bleeding and others. Overall, the evidence-based literature focuses on managing pain symptomatically according to its etiology.

- Primary and secondary lymphedema manifestations are rarer on upper limbs compared to lower limbs.
- Solid tumors and radiation therapy increase the risk for upper limb lymphedema.
- Differential diagnosis for unilateral adult-onset upper limb lymphedema includes secondary lymphedema (systemic disease and occult malignancy). If ruled out, primary causes (e.g., lymphedema tarda) should be considered.
- Advanced imaging with LSG is considered the gold standard to confirm the diagnosis of lymphedema.
- Treatment of lymphedema is dependent on its stage and successful treatment of any underlying causative disease; therefore, treatment delays should be avoided.
- Evidence-based therapies for lymphedema include compressive decongestive therapy, exercises, and skin care/hygiene.
- Obesity and lack of exercise increase the risk of lymphedema. Lifestyle modifications should be prescribed throughout all stages of the condition and be considered during surgical planning.
- Common upper limb pain patterns associated with lymphedema include neuropathic pain (lancinating severe pain associated with affection of the lower trunk of the brachial plexus and dull aching pain more commonly associated with the upper trunk as seen post-radiation) as well as soft tissue involvement (web cords and thoracic outlet syndrome), malignancy (tumor recurrences), and chronic pain syndromes (musculoskeletal soft tissue or joints involvement).
- Ultimately, the comprehensive assessment of lymphedema is complex. It entails careful clinical examination, testing with labs/imaging, and surveying for psychological health and quality of life. A multimodal therapeutic approach is the pilar to achieve comprehensive care and best outcomes, including psychological health and mitigation of associated disability.

Further Reading

Borman P. Lymphedema diagnosis, treatment, and follow-up from the viewpoint of physical medicine and rehabilitation specialists. *Turk J Phys Med Rehabil.* 2018;64(3):179–197.

Fife CE, Farrow W, Herbert AA, et al. Skin and wound care in lymphedema patients: A taxonomy, primer, and literature review. *Adv Skin Wound Care.* 2017;30(7):305–318.

Forte AJ, Huayllani MT, Boczar D, Cinotto G, McLaughlin SA. Lipoaspiration and controlled compressive therapy in lymphedema of the upper extremity: A comprehensive systematic review. *Cureus.* 2019;11(9):e5787.

Hutchinson NA. Lymphedema & arm discomfort after breast cancer. *Conquer.* 2015;1(6). Retrieved May 2020 from https://conquer-magazine.com/issues/2015/vol-1-no-6-december-2015/281-lymphedema-arm-discomfort-after-breast-cancer

Zeltzer AA, Anzarut A, Hamdi M. A review of lymphedema for the hand and upper-extremity surgeon. *J Hand Surg.* 2018;43(11):1016–1025.

Index

For the benefit of digital users, indexed terms that span two pages (e.g., 52–53) may, on occasion, appear on only one of those pages.

Tables, figures, and boxes are indicated by *t*, *f*, and *b* following the page number

Kiloh–Nevin syndrome, 94–95
Kleinman test, 113*f*, 113

labral tears, 3–5
lacertus fibrosus, 94–97
laser therapy. *See* low-level laser therapy
lateral epicondyle, 68
lateral epicondylitis ("tennis elbow"), 68–69
  provocative tests in the diagnosis of,
    68–69, 70*t*
  treatment, 69–70, 71–72
ligament of Struthers compression, 99
ligaments, 112, 123, 128, 130,
    134–35, 136
  lunotriquetral (LT) ligament, 113–14
  scapholunate ligament (SLL)
    injury, 110–12
  transverse carpal ligament, 106
long thoracic nerve, lesions to, 45
long thoracic nerve damage, 45
long thoracic nerve palsy, 47*f*
low-level laser therapy (LLLT), 22, 162
lunotriquetral (LT) ligament, 113
lunotriquetral (LT) ligament
    injuries, 113–14
  treatment, 114
lymphedema, 155, 156–57
  assessment and diagnosis, 159–60
  etiologies, 157*t*, 158, 162, 163
  pain in, 163
  primary vs. secondary, 157*t*, 159
  risk factors, 161–63
  stages, 160–61, 161*t*
  treatment/management, 161*t*, 161–63
lymphography, 160
lymphoscintigraphy, radionuclide, 160

magnetic resonance imaging (MRI), 62,
    71, 103–4
  arthrography and, 19–21, 26
  brachial plexopathies and, 56–58

edema and, 19–21, 71
  rotator cuff (RC) tears and, 6, 12, 26
  tendons and, 12, 19–21
manipulation under anesthesia
    (MUA), 28–29
medial epicondyle, 68, 85
medial epicondylitis ("golfer's elbow" and
    "pitcher's elbow"), 68, 97
metacarpophalangeal (MCP) joints,
    133, 134*f*, 135, 137*f*, 138*f*, 141,
    145–47, 149
muscle relaxants, 37
myelomalacia, 62
myokymia, 57–58

neck pain, 12–13, 61
neoplastic brachial plexopathy (NBP), 52–
    57, 55*t*, 58
nerve entrapment, 105–6. *See also* ulnar
    nerve entrapment
neuritis. *See* idiopathic brachial neuritis
neuropathic pain, 52–55, 88–89
  medications for, 36–37, 38
neuropathies, 57–58, 163
  compression, 52–53
nonsteroidal anti-inflammatory drugs
    (NSAIDs), 13, 38
  for bursitis, 82

O'Brien test, 20*t*
occult fractures, 110, 120
occupational therapists (OTs), 69–70
olecranon bursitis, 79
osteoarthritis (OA), 123, 127
  carpometacarpal (CMC), 129–31
  of GH joint, 5–6, 7
  most common joints affected by,
    135*f*, 135
  vs. rheumatoid arthritis
    (RA), 135
osteopenia, 137*f*